CARLAT PUBLISHING

Treating Opioid Use Disorder

———

A Fact Book

Noah Capurso, MD, MHS

Editor-in-Chief, *The Carlat Addiction Treatment Report*
Associate Professor of Psychiatry; Director of Didactic Education, Psychiatry
Yale University School of Medicine, New Haven, CT

Talia Puzantian, PharmD, BCPP

Professor, Keck Graduate Institute School of Pharmacy
Claremont, CA

Daniel J. Carlat, MD

Publisher, Carlat Publishing
Associate Clinical Professor, Tufts University School of Medicine
Boston, MA

Published by Carlat Publishing, LLC
PO Box 626, Newburyport, MA 01950

CARLAT PUBLISHING

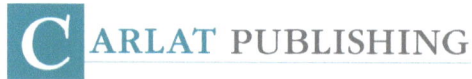

Published by Carlat Publishing, LLC
PO Box 626, Newburyport, MA 01950

Publisher and Editor-in-Chief: Daniel J. Carlat, MD
Deputy Editor: Talia Puzantian, PharmD, BCPP
Senior Editor: Ilana Fogelson
Associate Editor: Harmony Zambrano

This CME/CE activity is intended for psychiatrists, developmental and behavioral pediatricians, psychiatric nurses, psychologists, and other health care professionals, including primary care providers, with an interest in mental health. The Carlat CME Institute is accredited by the Accreditation Council for Continuing Medical Education to provide continuing medical education for physicians. The Carlat CME Institute maintains responsibility for this program and its content. The Carlat CME Institute designates this enduring material educational activity for a maximum of six (6) *AMA PRA Category 1 Credits*™. Physicians should claim credit commensurate only with the extent of their participation in the activity. CME quizzes must be taken online at www.thecarlatreport.com.

To order, visit www.thecarlatreport.com
or call (866) 348-9279

ISBN #:
Print - 979-8-9893264-0-2
eBook - 979-8-9893264-1-9

PRINTED IN THE UNITED STATES OF AMERICA

NOTES FROM THE AUTHORS

The goal of these fact sheets is to provide need-to-know information that can be easily and quickly absorbed and utilized during a busy day of seeing patients.

COST INFORMATION

We obtained pricing information for a one-month supply of a common dosing regimen from the website GoodRx (www.goodrx.com), accessed in October 2023. These are the prices patients would have to pay if they had no insurance (GoodRx also offers coupons to purchase certain medications at reduced prices). Because of wide variations in price depending on the pharmacy, we list price categories rather than the price in dollars. The categories are: $: Inexpensive (<$50/month); $$: Moderately expensive ($50–$100/month); $$$: Expensive ($100–$200/month); $$$$: Very expensive ($200–$500/month); $$$$$: Extremely expensive ($500/month).

FINANCIAL DISCLOSURES

Dr. Carlat, Dr. Capurso, and Dr. Puzantian have disclosed that they have no relevant relationships or financial interests in any commercial company pertaining to the information provided in this book.

DISCLAIMER

The information in this book was formulated with a reasonable standard of care and in conformity with current professional standards in the field of psychiatry. Treatment decisions are complex, and you should use these fact sheets as only one of many possible sources of medical information. Please refer to the *PDR (Physicians' Desk Reference)* when you need more in-depth information on medications. The information is not a substitute for informed medical care. This book is intended for use by licensed professionals only.

If you have any comments or corrections, please let us know by writing to us at info@thecarlatreport.com or The Carlat Psychiatry Report, P.O. Box 626, Newburyport, MA 01950.

Table of Contents

Opioid Use Disorder Overview

Opioids: The Basics of Street Drugs

Introduction

The global supply of illicit opioids is rapidly shifting and unstable. Fentanyl went from being an occasional contaminant to nearly completely taking over street opioids in the span of just a few years. More often than not, patients obtain different opioid drugs from a variety of sources. Depending on what is available at a given time, the same person may be sniffing, smoking, injecting, or swallowing different varieties of opioids, some illegal (such as heroin), some legal but illicitly obtained (such as OxyContin), and some legal drugs that were manufactured illicitly (such as fentanyl). In this fact sheet, we introduce you to the landscape of street opioids in order to help you understand what your patients are using and allow you to speak their language.

Heroin

- *Basics:* A prodrug of morphine, heroin is a natural product manufactured from poppy plants most commonly grown in Southern Asia and Central America. For decades, it was the dominant illicit opioid available on the street, until it was overtaken by fentanyl in recent years. Heroin can come in various forms, most commonly a white powder, a brown powder, or a black sticky substance called "black tar."
- *Street names:* Dope, H, smack, junk, snow, China white, black tar, brown; also known as speed ball when mixed with cocaine.
- *How it's obtained:* Street dealers sell heroin in small plastic or paper bags, each of which is supposed to contain a single dose. The actual amount of heroin per bag varies from as little as 25 mg to as much as 100 mg. Ten bags make up a "bundle," and five bundles make up a "brick."
- *How it's used:* Injected, smoked, sniffed, or administered subcutaneously ("skin popping").
- *Cost:* One bag typically costs $10–$20.
- *Average daily use:* Varies significantly, but a typical daily dose for someone who uses heroin might be 100–500 mg or more, divided into multiple doses throughout the day.

Fentanyl

- *Basics:* Fentanyl is a powerful synthetic opioid commonly used for the treatment of perioperative and chronic pain. When sold on the street, however, it is rarely pharmaceutical-grade medication. Instead, it is an illegally manufactured product, usually from China, that is smuggled into the country. Quality control is very poor—thus "fentanyl" often contains impurities and can be mixed with highly potent structural analogues such as carfentanil and sufentanil. Illicit fentanyl has nearly completely overtaken the drug market—it is found in almost all illicit opioids and as contaminants in non-opioid drugs like cocaine and amphetamines.
- *Street names:* Crazy one, dragon's breath, great bear, goodfella, poison.
- *How it's obtained:* Typically sold in the same manner as heroin (in single-dose bags) or as counterfeit pills.
- *How it's used:* Pharmaceutical fentanyl can be taken intravenously, as a transdermal patch (which is sometimes chewed or smoked), and as a lozenge. Illicit fentanyl is used intravenously, sniffed, swallowed, or smoked.
- *Cost:* A 2020 study found that prices for fentanyl are 10–20 times cheaper than heroin (Broadhurst R et al, *Trends and Issues in Crime and Criminal Justice* 2020;590:1–14), which explains its rise in the illicit marketplace. Bags of fentanyl are sold for a few dollars apiece; patches cost approximately $50 apiece.
- *Average daily use:* Difficult to estimate, but a typical user might use 50–200 mcg or more, divided into multiple doses throughout the day.

Oxycodone/OxyContin/Percocet

- *Basics:* OxyContin, the long-acting formulation of oxycodone, is a semi-synthetic prescription opioid introduced in 1996. The high doses contained within a single pill, intranasal bioavailability, and aggressive marketing campaign have been cited as supercharging the "first wave" of the opioid epidemic. Cheap and widely available heroin eventually replaced OxyContin as the main driver of opioid-related morbidity and mortality in the late 2000s once prescriptions were dialed back. Oxycodone and OxyContin are less commonly seen on the streets these days, though they are still available. Percocet is branded oxycodone co-formulated with acetaminophen.
- *Street names:* Oxy, roxy, OC, greenies, perc, hillbilly heroin.
- *How it's obtained:* Tablets on the street originate from one of two sources. Some are actual pharmaceutical-grade tablets. Others are counterfeits. These "pressed pills" can be nearly indistinguishable from the real thing but contain dangerous amounts of contaminants, often fentanyl or fentanyl analogues.
- *How it's used:* Swallowed or sniffed.
- *Cost:* Individual tablets sell for $5–$20 apiece or more.

- *Average daily use:* A typical daily dose for an oxycodone user might be 20–240 mg or more, divided into multiple doses throughout the day.

Other Prescription Opioids

- *Basics:* Although OxyContin has been assigned much of the blame for driving the early opioid epidemic, other prescription opioid analgesics had a part to play as well. Fentanyl is more commonly found on the streets, but various opioid analgesics can still be purchased. The specific agents available vary by geography and tend to shift over time, but as with OxyContin, counterfeit "pressed pills" containing potentially lethal doses of fentanyl remain a constant danger.
- *Specific agents:*
  - Hydromorphone (Dilaudid, Exalgo): known as smack, juice, D, dillies, footballs.
  - Hydrocodone/acetaminophen (Vicodin): known as vikes, hydro, banana, fluff.
  - Oxymorphone (Opana): known as Mrs. O, O-bomb, octagon, biscuits.
  - Morphine (MS Contin): known as morpho, M, Miss Emma, monkey.
  - Codeine/acetaminophen (Tylenol #3, Tylenol #4): known as T3, T4.
  - Codeine: known as Cody, Captain Cody, little C.
  - Codeine/promethazine syrup (typically mixed with soda): known as purple drank, Texas tea, sizzurp.
  - Meperidine (Demerol): known as demmies, dillies, D.
- *How they're used:* Typically swallowed or sniffed.
- *Cost:* Varies by agent and geographic region, anywhere from a few dollars to $50+ per dose.

Xylazine

Introduction
The illicit opioid supply has become increasingly unpredictable. Over the last 10 years, fentanyl and its derivatives have found their way into this supply and have become key contributors to the continued increase in overdose deaths. One of the most concerning and persistent additives is xylazine, known on the street as "tranq." Here, we will cover the basic pharmacology of xylazine, why it's so concerning, what to look out for if you suspect it, and how to counsel your patients.

What Is Xylazine?
Xylazine is a non-opioid veterinary anesthetic not approved for human consumption. However, it has been illicitly combined with opioids. Some believe that xylazine is added to opioids to enhance and prolong their sedative and euphoric effects.

- *Usage method:* Xylazine is available in liquid and powder form, although it is rarely used on its own. It is almost always combined with opioids that can be injected, smoked, or sniffed. Some seek out xylazine for its sedating effects, though usage is often inadvertent, as xylazine is usually added to opioids without the knowledge of the person buying and using the drug.
- *Mechanism of action:* Predominantly acts as an alpha-2 agonist.
- *Duration of effects:* The profound sedation caused by xylazine, especially in synergy with opioids, can last for hours.
- *Elimination rate:* While fentanyl has a short half-life and is quickly eliminated, xylazine's effects last longer. People often wake up after using xylazine already in opioid withdrawal and with powerful cravings to use again.
- *Testing:* Xylazine test strips have been developed and are available to the public through harm reduction programs.
- *History:* Xylazine first tainted the opioid supply in the early 2000s in Puerto Rico. Philadelphia, Pennsylvania, has become a major distribution hub, with nearly all street-sold opioids there containing xylazine. Although it's most commonly found in the Northeast, xylazine has been detected in the drug supply throughout the US with growing prevalence.

Why Should We Be Concerned?
- *Synergistic sedative effects:* When combined with opioids, xylazine produces profound sedation, increasing the risks to the user for becoming a victim of theft or physical and/or sexual assault.
- *Health risks:* Xylazine causes significant hypotension and bradycardia, and the resulting drop in blood flow can lead to loss of consciousness and hypoperfusion. Unlike overdoses due to opioids, there are no antidotes to reverse xylazine toxicity.
- *Wound complications:* Repeated exposure to xylazine causes severe peripheral wounds—usually in extremities, sometimes far from the site of injection. Wounds can become ulcerated or necrotic, and require surgical debridement or even amputation. They may result from decreased perfusion and oxygenation secondary to the severe hypotension and bradycardia induced by xylazine.

Recommendations for Professionals
- *Treatment:* Treat opioid use disorder as xylazine is rarely used on its own and is usually mixed with opioids. Patients not using illicit opioids are unlikely to encounter xylazine.
- *Overdose handling:* Give naloxone in overdose situations. While it won't reverse xylazine's effects, it will reverse the overdose of any opioids that were also consumed.
- *Recognition:* Suspect xylazine intoxication when overdose victims are not fully revived after receiving naloxone. Provide supportive care in the meantime while xylazine is eliminated from the body.
- *Physical exam:* Do a thorough skin exam on patients using illicit opioids whenever possible and refer to wound care specialists if needed.

Counseling Patients
- *Awareness:* Make sure patients are aware of xylazine's dangers.
- *Drug testing:* Encourage your patients to check any opioid that they intend to use for the presence of xylazine using xylazine test strips. They are widely available for purchase and through some harm reduction organizations.
- *Self-inspection:* Encourage patients to check their own skin and seek care if they notice any wounds.
- *Usage method:* Intravenous use seems to cause worse wounds, so encourage patients who are actively using to switch their route of administration.
- *Preparedness:* Make sure your patients have naloxone available.

Overview of Treatment Options for Opioid Use Disorder

Introduction

As treatment options for patients with opioid use disorder (OUD) expand, it's important to have a handy overview available to guide your conversations with patients. In this fact sheet, we cover the most evidence-based treatments and provide guidance for how to choose among them.

Medication for Opioid Use Disorder (MOUD)

Previously known as medication-assisted treatment (MAT), MOUD is the gold standard treatment, and the only approach convincingly shown to decrease opioid overdose mortality as well as all-cause mortality. MOUD also increases treatment retention, reduces opioid use, and mitigates harms associated with use. Of the three MOUD medications, methadone and buprenorphine have by far the most robust evidence base, though injectable naltrexone is catching up.

Methadone

- Methadone is a long-acting opioid agonist that reduces withdrawal symptoms and cravings. Its long half-life means that it can be taken once daily, and its slow time of onset means that it doesn't cause the intense euphoric effects of other opioids. It can only be dispensed through a federally licensed opioid treatment program (OTP), commonly called a "methadone clinic," when used to treat OUD.
- *Most appropriate use:* Consider methadone for patients who still experience opioid cravings on buprenorphine and those who could benefit from the structure of an OTP.
- *Usual treatment procedure:* Patients can start methadone in a hospital or ER setting but must enroll in a federally licensed OTP to continue treatment. Doses cannot exceed 40 mg over the first 24 hours and are gradually increased over the course of several weeks.
- *Continuing treatment:* Because methadone is a full agonist, it does not have a physiologic ceiling effect and can therefore be increased until the patient no longer has opioid cravings. That's usually around 90 mg, but some patients require much higher doses.

Buprenorphine

- Buprenorphine is a partial opioid agonist that can be prescribed in an office-based setting. It can be dispensed as sublingual films, sublingual tablets, or a long-acting injectable. Sublingual forms are often combined with naloxone in order to deter intravenous use.
- *Most appropriate use:* Buprenorphine is a good first-line treatment for most patients with OUD given its robust evidence base, ease of use, and better accessibility than methadone.
- *Usual treatment procedure:* Because of its partial agonism property, taking a dose of buprenorphine with opioid agonists in the system can cause precipitated withdrawal. Therefore, buprenorphine is usually started once the patient is in moderate withdrawal, and the dose is increased over a few days, a procedure called "induction."
- *Continuing treatment:* Buprenorphine can be increased by 8 mg each day, up to a total daily dose of 24 mg. Because buprenorphine is a partial agonist, few patients will derive benefit from going above this dose. If the patient is still experiencing cravings at 24 mg daily, consider switching to methadone.

Naltrexone

- Naltrexone is an opioid antagonist that blocks the effects of opioids and decreases cravings. While it is available as a pill, only the extended-release monthly injection (Vivitrol) has been shown to be effective for OUD.
- *Most appropriate use:* Naltrexone can be tricky to start, so it is best reserved for those who start their treatment in a supervised setting, either inpatient, a residential treatment program, or a jail/prison. Injectable naltrexone also can be a good option for the unhoused.
- *Usual treatment procedure:* Patients must be completely opioid free before the first dose of naltrexone is administered. For most opioids, that means at least a week, but it can take longer if the patient is taking a long-acting opioid like methadone. If there is any doubt, a naloxone challenge test can let you know if a patient is ready for naltrexone.
- *Continuing treatment:* Injectable naltrexone is meant to be administered once every four weeks; however, this interval tends to be a bit long for some patients. You can give it at intervals as short as three weeks if your patient starts to develop drug cravings early.

Psychotherapy

Data have not shown psychosocial interventions to be an effective stand-alone treatment for OUD. However, they can be helpful for many patients when combined with MOUD.

Cognitive behavioral therapy (CBT)

- CBT is a psychotherapy that helps individuals identify and change negative thought patterns and behaviors. It can be delivered in individual or group settings.
- *Most appropriate use:* Individuals who are willing and able to complete homework assignments; patients with generally good follow-up.
- *Usual treatment procedure:* The first several sessions typically involve reviewing the fundamentals of CBT theory. Subsequent sessions are spent identifying negative thoughts, examining them, and restructuring them so that they cause less distress. Patients complete homework assignments that are then reviewed in session.

Contingency management (CM)

- CM is a behavioral therapy that provides incentives (eg, vouchers or prizes) for individuals to remain drug free. The most evidence for CM is in patients with stimulant use disorders. It can be delivered in individual or group settings.
- *Most appropriate use:* Patients enrolled in large treatment centers with CM research studies or grants to support such programs; those with comorbid stimulant use disorders.
- *Usual treatment procedure:* The first session is spent reviewing the structure and rules of the CM program that the patient is enrolling in. Patients will be screened for recent substance use during each visit, typically with a urine drug screen, and may be given access to a reward depending on the screen's results.

Motivational interviewing (MI)

- MI is a therapeutic approach that focuses on each patient's personal reasons for not using substances. It can be delivered in individual or group settings.
- *Most appropriate use:* Any patient. MI can be used in brief settings, like an ER, or longitudinally with established patients. It is particularly useful for patients who are reluctant to engage in treatment.
- *Usual treatment procedure:* Early sessions consist of building therapeutic rapport and agreeing upon a change goal. In later sessions, the therapist explores and enhances the patient's own reasons for sobriety and helps the patient construct a change plan.

Opioid Use Disorder Assessment

Opioid Use Disorder: How to Conduct the Initial Assessment

Initial Questions

As with any psychiatric interview, start by building an alliance and showing interest in your patient in a general way. The first few questions, although not explicitly related to psychiatric issues, will typically naturally transition to the patient's reason for their visit.

- "Where are you from?"
- "What do you do for work and fun?"

Core Questions

We suggest you ask some version of the following questions to every patient you evaluate with opioid use disorder. RIPTEAR is a useful mnemonic that gets you the information needed for both acute and long-term treatment planning (www.coursera.org/learn/addiction-treatment).

Risk—Assess for acute risks that might need immediate intervention, including current intoxication that could lead to overdose (nodding off, not responding), acute suicidality, or active medical issues.

- "You've been going through a lot recently; have you been having any thoughts of harming yourself?"
- "Do you have any medical issues that need to be addressed right away, such as infections at injection sites?"

Initiation—Learn when the patient started using opioids to give you an idea about the trajectory of their use disorder.

- "How old were you when you first started using?"
- "How old were you when you started using regularly?"
- "When did you recognize your use was a problem?"
- "What was your period of heaviest use?"

Pattern of use—Look into pattern of use to further understand the course of the patient's use disorder as well as get an idea of their level of tolerance and potential for specific consequences such as infections, overdose, and withdrawal.

- "What drugs are you using and how are you using them?"
- "How much have you been using lately?"
- "What might happen if you were to stop using?" (this gets at withdrawal)
- "Do you use with people or alone?" (using alone increases risk for fatal overdose)

Treatment—Get an idea of the patient's treatment history to help you collaborate with the patient and come up with a plan that is likely to work.

- "Tell me about treatment you've had in the past."
- "What treatments worked and what didn't work?"

Effects—Ask about the effects that opioids have in the patient's life, both positive and negative. Understanding the positive effects of opioids can help identify targets of treatment. Negative effects can serve as points of motivation for sobriety.

- "Help me understand what role drugs play in your life."
- "What do you get out of them?"
- "What sorts of problems do they cause for you?"

Abstinence—Find out if the patient has ever had significant periods of abstinence in their life and how they were able to achieve that.

- "Tell me about periods in your life when you were able to stay sober."
- "What was going on that allowed you to achieve sobriety?"

Return to use—Investigate the circumstances around return to use to help you and the patient look ahead to potential problems.

- "Have you ever had a return to use after a period of sobriety?"
- "What were the circumstances that led you to return to use?"
- "What might you be able to change in order to prevent that from happening again?"

Assessing Severity

While the DSM-5 has clear cutoff points for distinguishing mild, moderate, and severe disorder, the following will help you quickly identify typical patient scenarios that would fall into a given category.

Mild:

- Taking a low dose of a low-potency opioid (like codeine)
- Opioid use confined to prescription opioid analgesics, no use of heroin or illicit fentanyl
- Able to maintain a job, a relationship, and appearance of normal functioning

Moderate:

- Using opioids daily or nearly daily
- Has experienced withdrawal symptoms
- Some consequences due to their opioid use, such as having lost a significant relationship or even a job
- No opioid-related health problems

Severe:

- Using opioids multiple times throughout the day
- Develops severe withdrawal symptoms if they don't use
- Lost relationships with friends or family
- Spending significant amounts of money on opioids
- May have switched to intranasal or IV use to overcome effects of tolerance and reduce costs
- History of serious health consequences such as accidental overdose, abscesses at injection sites, or bloodborne infections such as HIV or hepatitis B or C

Opioid Use Disorder: Initial Evaluation Template

Introduction
This template can be downloaded and adapted for your charting, or you can use it as a guide to remind you of important topics to cover during the initial interview.

Identifying Data
- Name:
- Age:
- Demographic information:

History of Present Illness (Focused on Opioid Use)
Assessment of current opioid use:
- Type of opioid used: prescription pills (ask about source: pharmacy vs counterfeit), heroin, fentanyl
- Route of administration: intranasal ("sniffing," "snorting"), intravenous ("shooting," "mainlining"), subcutaneous ("skin popping")
- Amount used:
  - Prescription analgesics are typically described in milligrams.
  - Illicit opioids are quantified in "bags." Bag size can be 25–100 mg, and the purity of what the bag contains is variable. Ten bags = 1 "bundle." Use of >1 bundle a day is heavy use. Five bundles or 50 bags = 1 "brick."
- Frequency of use: most common is 2–6 times daily
- Duration of most recent period of use
- Time of most recent use

Assessment of prior opioid use:
- Age of first use
- Total duration of use
- Period of heaviest use
- History of overdose
- History of hospitalization
- History of receiving naloxone

Negative consequences of opioid use:
- Medical consequences:
- Social or interpersonal problems:
- Impaired ability to fulfill role obligations (work, school, home):
- Overdose history:

Treatment history:
- Medications for opioid use disorder (MOUD) (buprenorphine, methadone, naltrexone)
- Rehabilitation/residential treatment
- 12-step program participation
- Individual and/or group therapy
- Sober housing
- How long was the longest period of sobriety? How was the patient able to achieve that?
- What treatments worked and why? What treatments didn't work and why?

Other substance use history:
- Other substances the patient uses, severity of use, and treatment history

Past Psychiatric History (Non-Substance Use Disorders)
- Previous psychiatric diagnoses
- Past psychiatric medications
- Previous psychiatric hospitalizations
- Suicidal ideation, prior attempts (especially if an attempt involved opioids)

Medical History

Assessment of comorbid medical conditions:

- Respiratory conditions, such as COPD and sleep apnea, can increase risk of overdose
- Cardiac conditions can limit treatment options (ie, methadone)
- Liver and renal disease can impact drug metabolism and could require dosing adjustments
- Infectious diseases, such as skin infections, HIV, hepatitis B, or hepatitis C, may require some integrated care
- Comorbid pain conditions could make treatment challenging and could necessitate referral to a pain specialist
- Obtain a current medication list, paying particular attention to CNS depressants and medications that can interact with MOUDs

Social History

Assess the patient's living situation: homelessness, access to transportation, ability to regularly access treatment, potential work conflicts, what treatments they can afford.

Mental Status Exam

Pay particular attention to signs of opioid intoxication (slurred speech, slowed cognition, drowsiness) and opioid withdrawal (anxiety, irritability, appearing "sick").

Labs

- *Basic labs:* complete blood count, electrolyte panel, kidney function, liver function
- *Transmissible disease panel:* HIV antibody, syphilis, tuberculosis (skin test or QuantiFERON), hepatitis B (HBsAg, anti-HBs, anti-HBc), and hepatitis C (antibody with reflex HCV RNA test)
- *Urine drug screening:* fentanyl and methadone may need to be added separately; consider confirmatory testing for positive or otherwise suspicious results

Assessment and Plan

Pharmacological interventions:

- If buprenorphine, lay out induction plan (home vs clinic vs inpatient). Is the patient in sufficient withdrawal now to proceed with induction? Is microdosing preferred?
- If methadone, where might the patient follow up?
- If injectable naltrexone, when will the patient be ready for the first dose? Who will administer it and where?

Other psychotherapeutic services, social support/resources:

- Referral to psychotherapy?
- Social services (including housing assistance, supportive employment, food assistance, legal services)?

Follow-up plan:

- Date of next follow-up:
- Specify modalities (face to face vs telehealth):

How to Ask DSM-5 Focused Questions for Opioid Use Disorder

Introduction

Like all substance use disorders, opioid use disorder (OUD), defined by the DSM-5, includes 11 criteria. While most experienced clinicians can diagnose OUD without going through a formal checklist of symptoms, we suggest you try using this sheet during interviews. You are likely to find it helpful in at least two ways.

First, you can use the criteria to more accurately categorize the severity of your patient's OUD:

- Mild: two to three DSM-5 criteria
- Moderate: four to five DSM-5 criteria
- Severe: more than five DSM-5 criteria

Second, you can use the criteria to show your patient that there are objective symptoms leading to the diagnosis of OUD. This may lessen the stigma attached to the diagnosis and help your patient identify with the diagnosis and invest in treatment.

Below, we suggest questions for each of the 11 criteria. Although the DSM-5 doesn't explicitly divide the criteria into categories, we find it helpful to do so, and below we list them under four broad clusters: impairment of control, social consequences, risky behavior, and tolerance/withdrawal.

Questions About Time Spent Obtaining Opioids (Impairment of Control)

Cravings:
- "Do you have cravings (urges to use opioids)?"

Using more than planned:
- "Do you often use more opioids than you really want to or intend to?"

Unable to quit despite attempts to do so:
- "Have you tried to cut down or quit using opioids before?"
- "What is the longest time you have been abstinent? How long ago was that?"

Significant time spent obtaining or recovering from opioids:
- "How often do you go to the pharmacy or dealer?"
- "How long do you spend using opioids?"
- "How many hours per day do you avoid family or work because of using opioids or recovering from their effects?"

Questions About Activities Given Up Over Time Due to Opioid Use (Social Consequences)

1. *Activities given up due to opioid use:* "Are you spending less time with your family than before?" "Have you avoided going out because you are at home using opioids instead?"
2. *Failure to fulfill major role obligations:* "Have you had to take time off from work or call in sick because of opioid use?"
3. *Persistent social and interpersonal problems:* "How much time do you spend socializing in settings that don't involve opioids? Is this less time than before?" "Do you have arguments with friends or family over opioid use?" "Have you lost contact with friends due to opioid use?"

Questions About Use in Hazardous Situations (Risky Behavior)

4. *Recurrent use in physically hazardous situations:* "Have you ever used opioids while driving or operating heavy machinery?" "Have you ever used opioids while on the job?"
5. *Continued use despite knowledge of negative consequences:* "Have you continued to use opioids after hearing from a doctor about medical problems caused by opioid use or learning about the risk of overdose?" "Have you continued to use opioids after experiencing any personal or medical problems, including overdose, caused by opioid use?"

Questions About Tolerance and Withdrawal

6. *Tolerance:* "Do you need to use more opioids than you previously did to achieve the same effect?"
7. *Withdrawal:* "Have you been through opioid withdrawal before?" "Do you experience opioid withdrawal symptoms between doses?" "Have you had problems with sleep, mood, or physical symptoms after stopping or reducing opioid use?"

Medical Issues and Opioid Use Disorder

Introduction

While you may not be treating most medical complications of opioid use disorder, any comprehensive assessment of these patients should include a screening for the most common medical complications.

Common Opioid-Related Medical Issues

Transmissible viral infections

- *Hepatitis B:* Spread by contact with infected blood or semen, so sharing needles and sexual contact are both common ways of contracting it. The acute phase of the illness usually occurs within two weeks of contact and causes symptoms that may seem like the flu, such as fever, joint pain, fatigue, and sometimes jaundice. Hepatitis B can become a chronic infection, though this only occurs in 5% of adults who contract the virus. There is a vaccine to prevent hepatitis B, but unlike hepatitis C, there are no curative treatments. Patients will typically be followed by a specialist for years, with lab monitoring every six to 12 months. Patients with chronic hepatitis B will be asymptomatic for most of their lives, but about 10% will develop liver cancer or cirrhosis, which has a high mortality rate.

- *Hepatitis C:* Spread by contact with infected blood, most commonly through sharing needles. It can be transmitted through sexual contact and sharing of drug sniffing implements as well, though the incidence is low. Acute infection is mild and usually asymptomatic, but it is much more likely than hepatitis B to become a chronic infection, with 75% of patients developing chronic hepatitis C. Chronic hepatitis C is a major cause of liver cirrhosis, cancer, and eventual transplantation. However, unlike hepatitis B, there are now several treatments with a 90% or better cure rate. These are often combination pills, such as ledipasvir/sofosbuvir (Harvoni) and elbasvir/grazoprevir (Zepatier), and treatment usually lasts 12–24 weeks. There is no vaccine to prevent hepatitis C.

- *HIV:* Spread through sexual contact or contact with infected blood, typically by sharing needles. About half of patients who contract the virus develop flu-like symptoms within a month. Other patients are initially asymptomatic. There is no vaccine and no cure, though patients can live for many years with HIV while taking highly active anti-retroviral therapy (HAART). Transmission can be greatly reduced with pre- and post-exposure prophylaxis (see "Harm Reduction and Opioid Use Disorder" fact sheet).

Sequelae of intravenous (IV) use

- *Track marks:* IV use over time results in track marks, thin lines of callus-like skin that follow the course of a vein.
- *Bacterial infection:* Injection of drugs carries high risk for bacterial infection.
- *Cellulitis and skin abscess:* Exam reveals painful red, purple, or black skin, often with a collection of pus. Requires antibiotics, and some patients need hospitalization for IV antibiotics or surgical debridement. Opioids that have been adulterated with xylazine are particularly associated with dangerous soft tissue wounds (see "Xylazine" fact sheet).
- *Endocarditis:* Usually right sided. Patients will have fever, malaise, weight loss, and other nonspecific symptoms. Septic emboli to the lungs cause cough, dyspnea, and pleuritic chest pain. Heart murmur may be heard on physical exam, though not always. Definitive test is blood culture and echocardiogram. Refer to cardiology if you have any suspicion of endocarditis.
- *Osteomyelitis:* Most often in the area of the sternum. Symptoms include localized pain in the anterior chest, and exam reveals swelling of the chest or a tender mass over the sternum. Labs reveal elevated ESR and CRP. Refer to a specialist for imaging and possible biopsy if you suspect osteomyelitis.
- *Constipation:* Chronic opioid use can cause severe constipation. Many patients will have only a couple of bowel movements a week. Treat constipation with an aggressive bowel regimen, and avoid bulk-forming agents like psyllium.

Issues surrounding surgery

- Patients with chronic exposure to opioids (illicit or prescribed) typically have a high tolerance to their analgesic effects. Tolerance to respiratory suppression is usually not nearly as developed, however. Many of these patients require higher than usual doses of opioids for pain control during and immediately after surgery, but they are at high risk of respiratory suppression. Monitor these patients closely!
- Patients on buprenorphine may need to adjust their medication before a major surgery. If this is the case, collaborate closely with the anesthesia and surgical teams. The general guidance is to stop buprenorphine the day before surgery and then resume the medication on postop day 1. Adjunctive opioid analgesic medication can be used sparingly on top of buprenorphine for a short time.

Labs to Consider Upon Intake/Initial Workup

- Transmissible infection panel
  - HIV antibody
  - Hepatitis B (HBsAg, anti-HBs, anti-HBc)
  - Hepatitis C (antibody with reflex HCV RNA test)
  - Tuberculosis if history of incarceration: tuberculin skin test (PPD) or QuantiFERON
  - Syphilis if history of high-risk sexual behaviors
- Chemistries
- Complete blood count (CBC): Elevated white count can be indicative of infection
- Liver function tests
  - Transaminases (AST and ALT): Elevations are caused by leakage from damaged liver cells. Mild elevations (less than four times the upper limit of normal) are common and usually reversible with abstinence. More concerning are elevations of four or more times the upper limit of normal (usually >200 depending on the lab).
  - Synthetic function: Increased bilirubin, increased INR, and decreased albumin indicate decreased synthetic function and imply pending liver failure
- ESR and CRP if there are symptoms consistent with osteomyelitis
- EKG if there is a history of cardiac disease or the patient is on other QT-prolonging agents
- Urine toxicology: Be sure to add fentanyl, buprenorphine, and methadone separately if they are not included at your institution

Opioid Withdrawal Management

Opioid Withdrawal Management

Introduction

Getting patients with opioid use disorder (OUD) completely off opioids, so-called "detox," is generally not advisable. Very few patients with OUD are able to completely stop opioids and remain abstinent for any length of time without further treatment. Moreover, taking patients off opioids completely can lower tolerance and paradoxically *increase* risk of overdose in the long run. The only situation in which medically supervised withdrawal is a sensible approach is if the patient plans to receive intramuscular naltrexone immediately afterwards, but even this approach can be tough outside of controlled inpatient settings.

Nonetheless, some patients will insist on getting off all opioids. For these patients, a medically supervised opioid withdrawal is preferable to no care at all. Contrary to popular belief, the vomiting, diarrhea, and autonomic instability that patients experience during opioid withdrawal can be fatal for those with underlying medical conditions that impact their ability to regulate fluid balance or those who are at risk of developing cardiac arrhythmias. Opioid withdrawal can be especially risky in pregnant patients since it can lead to fetal demise. Finally, easing the symptoms of withdrawal at the very least can help keep your patient engaged with treatment. Be sure to provide these patients with naloxone in the likely event they return to use, and make sure they know how to get treatment if they change their mind.

There are two general approaches. Opioid-assisted withdrawal management, with buprenorphine or methadone, is preferable because withdrawal is less severe (Meader N, *Drug Alcohol Depend* 2010;108(1–2):110–114). Symptom-based treatment with alpha-2 agonists and adjunctive medications should be used only when opioid medications are not available.

Inpatient vs Outpatient

Good Candidates for Outpatient	Candidates Who Need Inpatient*
Medically healthy	Medical comorbidities
Good social supports	Living alone, unhoused, or otherwise isolated
Reliable	History of poor follow-up
Cognitively intact	Cognitively impaired
Access to transportation	No reliable transportation
No active psychiatric illness	Unstable major mental illness
Buprenorphine or symptom-based protocol	Methadone protocol
	Pregnant

*See "Managing Opioid Withdrawal in the Inpatient Setting" fact sheet for more details

Opioid-Assisted Withdrawal Management

Buprenorphine has less risk of overdose and is therefore preferred over methadone. Remember, buprenorphine can worsen withdrawal if given too early, and methadone can stack with other opioids in the patient's system. Therefore, start treatment once the patient is in moderate withdrawal (a score of around 8 on the Clinical Opiate Withdrawal Scale [COWS] or a score of about 10 on the Subjective Opiate Withdrawal Scale [SOWS]). Give just enough medication to control withdrawal symptoms and taper over five days or so. Here are sample protocols, which should be adjusted based upon patient response.

	Buprenorphine	Methadone
Day 1	4 mg BID	5–10 mg Q2hrs up to 40 mg
Day 2	4 mg BID	30 mg daily
Day 3	3 mg BID	20 mg daily
Day 4	2 mg BID	10 mg daily
Day 5	1 mg BID	5 mg daily

Symptom-Based Treatment

Alpha-2 agonists can relieve autonomic symptoms of opioid withdrawal like GI distress, anxiety, sweating, and cramping. They cause hypotension as a side effect, so be sure to check blood pressure before each dose and hold the dose if SBP<90 or DBP<60. If outpatient, have patients check blood pressure before taking a dose. Consider the following adjunctive medications as well:

Symptom	Medication	Notes
Autonomic symptoms	Clonidine: 0.1–0.2 mg Q1hr; max 0.8 mg/day Lofexidine: 0.54 mg Q6hrs; max 2.88 mg/day	Give 0.1 mg if COWS or SOWS<12 Give 0.2 mg if COWS or SOWS>12 Take total dose in the first 24 hours; give in divided doses QID for several days; taper 0.1–0.2 mg/day until discontinuation (slow taper avoids rebound hypertension)
Anxiety	Hydroxyzine: 25–50 mg Q6hrs; max 200 mg/day Lorazepam: 1 mg Q4–6hrs; max 4 mg/day	Reserve benzos for inpatient Avoid benzos if patient takes other CNS depressants
Nausea/vomiting	Ondansetron: 4 mg Q4–6hrs; max 16 mg/day Prochlorperazine: 5 mg QID; max 20 mg/day	Prochlorperazine is an antipsychotic and can help relieve anxiety, though risks akathisia as well
Diarrhea	Loperamide: 4 mg first, then 2 mg after each loose stool; max 16 mg/day	
Abdominal cramps	Dicyclomine: 10–20 mg Q6hrs	
Pain and muscle aches	Ibuprofen: 400–600 mg Q6hrs; max 2400 mg/day Acetaminophen: 650–1000 mg Q8hrs; max 3000 mg/day Naproxen: 500 mg BID	Steer clear of opioid analgesics, including tramadol
Insomnia	Trazodone: 25–100 mg QHS Quetiapine: 25–100 mg QHS	Reserve benzos and z-drugs for inpatient
Muscle spasm	Methocarbamol: 750–1500 mg Q8hrs Cyclobenzaprine: 5–10 mg Q6hrs; max 30 mg/day	

Patients receiving opioid-assisted withdrawal management may also benefit from the addition of adjunctive medications for symptom-based treatment as "comfort meds."

Opioid Withdrawal: Time Course and Symptoms

Who Is Likely to Experience Withdrawal Symptoms?
- It's hard to predict whether a particular person will experience withdrawal or how severe their symptoms will be. Generally speaking, **anyone who consistently takes an opioid for two weeks or longer is at risk**.
- Factors predicting **more severe withdrawal** include:
  - More consistent use (eg, every day as opposed to a few times a week)
  - Higher quantities used
  - Shorter-acting opioids (eg, two weeks of daily hydrocodone use will likely lead to worse withdrawal than two weeks of daily methadone use)
- Naloxone (Narcan) or naltrexone (Vivitrol) can trigger immediate (precipitated) withdrawal if given to someone who has opioids in their system.

What Are Common Opioid Withdrawal Symptoms?
- Mnemonic for remembering opioid withdrawal symptoms: **FLU OPRS**
  - **F**lu-like symptoms: Fever, sweating, and chills
  - **L**eg movements: Restless legs, kicking movements
  - **U**nwell feeling: General malaise or feeling unwell
  - **O**veractive reflexes: Twitching or spasms
  - **P**ain: Muscle aches, stomach cramping, and bone pain
  - **R**uns: Diarrhea and other gastrointestinal symptoms
  - **S**leep problems: Insomnia

When Does Withdrawal Begin and How Long Does It Last?
- Withdrawal usually starts after two or three half-lives of whatever opioid was used. The chart below is a rough guide for the expected time course of withdrawal; individual courses can be highly variable.

Drug	Withdrawal Onset	Peak of Withdrawal Symptoms	Duration of Withdrawal Syndrome
Fentanyl	3–12 hours	12–36 hours	5–7 days
Heroin	8–24 hours	36–72 hours	7–10 days
Short-acting analgesics (oxycodone, hydrocodone, morphine)	6–12 hours	12–36 hours	5–7 days
Long-acting analgesics (OxyContin, MS Contin, Opana)	8–24 hours	36–72 hours	7–10 days
Buprenorphine	1–2 days	3–5 days	10–20 days
Methadone	1–3 days	4–7 days	2–4 weeks

How Can You Measure Severity of Withdrawal?
- The **Clinical Opiate Withdrawal Scale (COWS)** is an 11-item clinician-administered scale that can be used in inpatient or outpatient settings. Its most common usage is to determine when a patient is ready for buprenorphine induction.
- The **Subjective Opiate Withdrawal Scale (SOWS)** is a self-administered version of the COWS that patients undergoing home induction can use to measure degree of withdrawal.

Practical Tips for Using the Clinical Opiate Withdrawal Scale (COWS)

Introduction

The Clinical Opiate Withdrawal Scale (COWS) is an 11-item scale used for rating the degree of opioid withdrawal. See our accompanying fact sheet that reproduces the entire scale for your use. While the COWS may appear straightforward, it can be confusing when using it to assess patients undergoing withdrawal in the real world. In this fact sheet, we offer some hard-won tips and pitfalls to avoid so that you can more accurately rate your patient's withdrawal symptoms.

Tips

1. *Familiarize yourself with the scale beforehand:* None of the symptoms are particularly difficult to evaluate on their own, but it is helpful to know how to rank each symptom before assessing a patient. Understanding the symptoms and their corresponding severity scores as listed on the COWS can help you make more accurate and consistent evaluations.

2. *Don't get vital signs right away:* Unlike the familiar Clinical Institute Withdrawal Assessment (CIWA) scale for alcohol withdrawal, COWS includes vital signs. We suggest measuring the vital signs toward the end of the assessment rather than at the beginning. This way, the patient will have been sitting for a few minutes (less than a minute of walking can elevate blood pressure and heart rate in some patients) and have had a chance for any potential anxiety to diminish.

3. *Establish a baseline:* Before treating withdrawal, obtain a baseline COWS score. This will allow you to track the patient's progress and response to treatment.

4. *Conduct assessments at regular intervals:* Use the COWS consistently at predetermined intervals (eg, every four to six hours) to monitor the patient's withdrawal symptoms. Regular measurements will help paint a picture of how the withdrawal syndrome is evolving so that you can make informed decisions about treatment and adjust on the fly if necessary.

5. *Combine with clinical judgment:* Although the COWS is a helpful tool, it does not take individual patient characteristics into account. For example, someone with an anxiety disorder might have an elevated heart rate regardless of their opioid withdrawal severity. Always integrate the results of the COWS with your clinical judgment, considering the patient's overall health and individual circumstances.

6. *Involve the patient:* Many of your patients will have gone through opioid withdrawal many times before. Their subjective report can be just as illuminating as the COWS. Encourage them to report any symptoms, and take these into consideration along with the COWS score when coming up with a treatment plan. If this is their first withdrawal, educate them about what to expect to facilitate open communication and collaboration.

Potential Pitfalls

1. *Overreliance on the scale:* Do not solely rely on the COWS for decision-making, as it is only one aspect of the patient's overall assessment. Always consider the patient's medical history, psychiatric history, concurrent medications, and comorbidities.

2. *Subjective scoring:* Some symptoms on the COWS might be challenging to assess objectively, such as anxiety or GI upset. Be cautious of potential biases when evaluating these symptoms and adhere to the descriptions on the scale as best you can.

3. *Inconsistent assessments:* Inaccurate results may occur if the COWS is not applied consistently or if different health care providers evaluate the patient without standardized criteria. Establish clear guidelines and promote inter-rater reliability. Again, adhering to the clinical descriptions on the scale itself can be helpful here.

4. *Misinterpretation of symptoms:* Some symptoms of opioid withdrawal may overlap with other medical conditions, such as anxiety disorders or GI issues. Carefully evaluate the patient's history and context to avoid misdiagnosis.

5. *Overlooking other medications and substances:* Prescription medications and non-opioid drugs can complicate the clinical picture. For instance, a beta-blocker can prevent rapid heart rate whereas a stimulant, prescribed or otherwise, might have the opposite effect. Be sure to get an accurate med list and substance use history and use this information when interpreting the COWS.

Clinical Opiate Withdrawal Scale

Introduction

The Clinical Opiate Withdrawal Scale (COWS) is an 11-item scale designed to be administered by a clinician. This tool can be used in both inpatient and outpatient settings to reproducibly rate common signs and symptoms of opiate withdrawal and monitor these symptoms over time. The summed score for the complete scale can be used to help clinicians determine the severity of opiate withdrawal.

Instructions

For each item, circle the number that best describes the patient's signs or symptoms. Rate based on your best judgment of an apparent relationship of a symptom to opiate withdrawal. For example, if heart rate is increased because the patient was jogging just prior to assessment, the increased pulse rate would not add to the score.

Patient's Name: _____   Date and Time _____

Reason for this assessment:_____

Resting Pulse Rate: _____ beats/minute *Measured after patient is sitting or lying for one minute* 0 pulse rate 80 or below 1 pulse rate 81–100 2 pulse rate 101–120 4 pulse rate greater than 120	**GI Upset:** *over last 1/2 hour* 0 no GI symptoms 1 stomach cramps 2 nausea or loose stool 3 vomiting or diarrhea 5 multiple episodes of diarrhea or vomiting
Sweating: *over past 1/2 hour not accounted for by room temperature or patient activity* 0 no report of chills or flushing 1 subjective report of chills or flushing 2 flushed or observable moistness on face 3 beads of sweat on brow or face 4 sweat streaming off face	**Tremor:** *observation of outstretched hands* 0 no tremor 1 tremor can be felt, but not observed 2 slight tremor observable 4 gross tremor or muscle twitching
Restlessness: *observation during assessment* 0 able to sit still 1 reports difficulty sitting still, but is able to do so 3 frequent shifting or extraneous movements of legs/arms 5 unable to sit still for more than a few seconds	**Yawning:** *observation during assessment* 0 no yawning 1 yawning once or twice during assessment 2 yawning three or more times during assessment 4 yawning several times/minute
Pupil Size 0 pupils pinned or normal size for room light 1 pupils possibly larger than normal for room light 2 pupils moderately dilated 5 pupils so dilated that only the rim of the iris is visible	**Anxiety or Irritability** 0 none 1 patient reports increasing irritability or anxiousness 2 patient obviously irritable or anxious 4 patient so irritable or anxious that participation in the assessment is difficult
Bone or Joint Aches: *if patient was having pain previously, only the additional component attributed to opiate withdrawal is scored* 0 not present 1 mild diffuse discomfort 2 patient reports severe diffuse aching of joints/muscles 4 patient is rubbing joints or muscles and is unable to sit still because of discomfort	**Gooseflesh Skin** 0 skin is smooth 3 piloerection of skin can be felt or hairs standing up on arms 5 prominent piloerection
Runny Nose or Tearing: *not accounted for by cold symptoms or allergies* 0 not present 1 nasal stuffiness or unusually moist eyes 2 nose running or tearing 4 nose constantly running or tears streaming down cheeks	**Total Score** _____ The total score is the sum of all 11 items Initials of person completing assessment: _____ Score: 5–12 = mild; 13–24 = moderate; 25–36 = moderately severe; more than 36 = severe withdrawal. This version may be copied and used clinically.

Source: Wesson DR and Ling W, *J Psychoactive Drugs* 2003;35(2):253–259.

Opioid Use Disorder Treatment: Medication

How to Choose the Right Medications for Opioid Use Disorder

Introduction

The purpose of this fact sheet is not to provide details on pharmacology or the use of these medications, but rather to help you decide which might be best for a given patient. For more detailed information on each agent, see the appropriate medication fact sheet.

Buprenorphine (Subutex) or Buprenorphine/Naloxone (Suboxone)

Buprenorphine is considered first line. Unlike methadone, you can prescribe it from a standard office setting and write for a month at a time. As a partial agonist, its ceiling effect makes overdose on buprenorphine alone unlikely. It is easier to initiate than naltrexone, which requires a period of abstinence, and can be quickly increased to therapeutic dose, whereas methadone can require a lengthy titration period.

There are two formulations of buprenorphine: buprenorphine monoproduct and buprenorphine/naloxone combination. The idea of the naloxone co-formulation is that it deters diversion or misuse by injection, but this isn't an absolute. Because there's less stigma attached to the co-formulation and it's much more broadly available, it's the favored formulation. Some may use the monoproduct during pregnancy to reduce medication exposure.

Best for: Most patients

Methadone

Methadone, for now, can only be prescribed at federally licensed opioid treatment programs (OTP)—colloquially known as "methadone clinics." Patients initially must show up six days per week to receive their dose and attend individual counseling sessions at least twice per month, or go to weekly group sessions. Clinic visits can be spaced out with "take-home privileges" after a period of stability, but intervals are rarely more than weekly. "Guest dosing" can be arranged at other OTPs when the patients travel, though this needs to be set up ahead of time.

Best for:
- Patients who benefit from increased structure—that is, observed dosing and daily monitoring. This includes patients who have had multiple accidental overdoses, those who have diverted their meds, and those with severe psychiatric or medical problems.
- Underserved and uninsured patients. Since methadone clinics are often publicly funded, patients will pay less out of pocket.
- Patients who continue to experience opioid cravings even on the maximum dose of buprenorphine (24–32 mg). The partial agonism of buprenorphine may not be sufficient for patients who have a very high tolerance. This may result from a history of using large amounts of high-potency opioids, typically fentanyl. As a full agonist, methadone has no ceiling effect, so the dose can be raised as high as needed to prevent cravings.

Naltrexone Monthly Injections (Vivitrol)

Vivitrol is a long-acting injectable form of naltrexone, which is an opioid receptor blocker like naloxone. It has two clinical effects. First, it decreases cravings, similar to the way it works for alcohol use disorder. Second, it blocks the effects of opioids if they are consumed within four weeks of administration, creating a behavioral incentive not to use opioids. Its biggest drawback is that it can only be given to patients who have been abstinent from opioids for a week (10–14 days for methadone).

Best for:
- Patients who have successfully gotten off all opioids and can remain abstinent from opioids for one week (that usually means an inpatient or residential setting).
- Unhoused patients—they do better on injectable naltrexone than buprenorphine, according to at least one study (Nunes EV Jr et al, *Am J Psychiatry* 2021;178(7):660–671).
- Patients who can't have any opioids in their system, typically due to workplace requirements (eg, health care workers, long-distance drivers, heavy machinery operators, etc).

How to Discuss and Initiate Buprenorphine

Introduction

Induction refers to the process of starting a patient on buprenorphine (with or without naloxone; the combination product is most often preferred). It can be done either inpatient or outpatient and typically takes two to three days, depending on the ultimate dose. See also the "Buprenorphine Microinduction" fact sheet for an alternative approach.

Step 1: Ensure Patient Is in Moderate Withdrawal Before the First Dose

Patients should stop opioids prior to induction and get their first dose of buprenorphine once in moderate withdrawal. Taking buprenorphine too soon can be very unpleasant, resulting in so-called "precipitated withdrawal." Depending on the opioid the patient is using, they could reach moderate withdrawal as soon as six hours or as long as several days after their last use.

For inpatient induction, patients are ready for their first dose when Clinical Opiate Withdrawal Scale scores reach 8 (see separate fact sheet). Dilated pupils are also a reliable sign. If at home, patients can score themselves with the Subjective Opiate Withdrawal Scale (see separate fact sheet); they're ready for buprenorphine once scores are between 8 and 10. They can also use the BUP Home Induction smartphone app, which can be downloaded free of charge through Apple's App Store or Google Play. Most patients with prior buprenorphine experience know when they're ready for a dose.

Step 2: Teach the Patient How to Take It

Most forms of buprenorphine are administered sublingually, and none of them should ever be swallowed; buprenorphine has poor oral bioavailability, so a swallowed tablet is a waste of money and can cause a stomachache. Sublingual tablets can take 10–15 minutes to dissolve; films take about a minute. First, tell patients to rinse their mouth out to get it nice and moist. Have them place the medication under their tongue and hold their tongue still until the medication is dissolved completely. The films can also be placed against the side of the cheek. Swallowing excess saliva is fine, but they should not talk. If they find the taste unpleasant, and most patients do, chewing up a sugar-free peppermint candy immediately before and after can be helpful. Patients should rinse their mouth out with water afterwards and avoid brushing their teeth for at least an hour.

Step 3: Give First Dose

A typical first dose of buprenorphine is 4 mg, though you can start with 2 mg for patients using small amounts of opioids (no more than two bags of heroin/fentanyl or less than 10 mg of oxycodone daily). If the patient still has withdrawal symptoms after one hour, give them an additional 4 mg. This is sufficient to relieve withdrawal symptoms in most patients. Some, especially those using large doses of fentanyl, may require a third 4 mg dose after another hour. The goal of the first day is to eliminate withdrawal.

Step 4: Optimize Dose

Once withdrawal symptoms are relieved, the goal becomes elimination of cravings. This usually requires a higher dose than the 8 or 12 mg from day 1. On the morning of day 2, the patient should take the total amount that was taken on day 1. If they still have opioid cravings, have them take another 4 or 8 mg, up to a total daily dose of 16 mg. Repeat on day 3 up to a total daily dose of 24 mg. Most patients will require 16–24 mg daily.

Step 5: Give Prescription and Schedule One-Week Follow-Up

Buprenorphine Induction Cheat Sheet

1. Patient must be in moderate withdrawal before their first dose of buprenorphine
2. Day 1: 4 mg doses of buprenorphine up to 12 mg; goal is to eliminate withdrawal symptoms
3. Day 2: Give first day's dose in the morning, then additional doses up to 16 mg; goal is to eliminate cravings
4. Day 3: Same as day 2, up to 24 mg; goal is to eliminate cravings
5. Once dose is finalized, make follow-up appointment for one week or less

---

Buprenorphine Microinduction

Rationale for Microinduction

The standard method of starting a patient on buprenorphine (see "How to Discuss and Initiate Buprenorphine" fact sheet) involves having the patient stop all opioids hours to days before the induction. This period is needed because buprenorphine can trigger opioid withdrawal if given when the patient still has most of their opioid receptors occupied by agonists. The downside to this standard induction method is that patients don't like having to experience withdrawal, even if it only scores as "moderate" on our rating scales.

In order to get around this, a newer induction strategy is gaining popularity, called microinduction (or microdosing). This involves introducing small amounts of buprenorphine and slowly increasing the dose while the patient remains on an opioid agonist. Once the buprenorphine dose is high enough to prevent withdrawal, typically 8–12 mg, the agonist is stopped. The idea is that no single dose increase is enough to cause discomfort.

Since the patient must remain on a full agonist for the duration of the microinduction, this strategy works best for patients on prescription opioids. While some clinicians are using microinduction to transition patients off of street opioids, we don't recommend it as a standard practice because microinduction takes longer than standard induction, leaving the patient undertreated and exposed to street opioids for longer than necessary. Microinduction is particularly well suited for methadone, whose long half-life can make inductions tricky. It's also appropriate for those who have previously failed a typical dosing initiation or are resistant to undergoing a withdrawal period. Here's a schematic of what's going on:

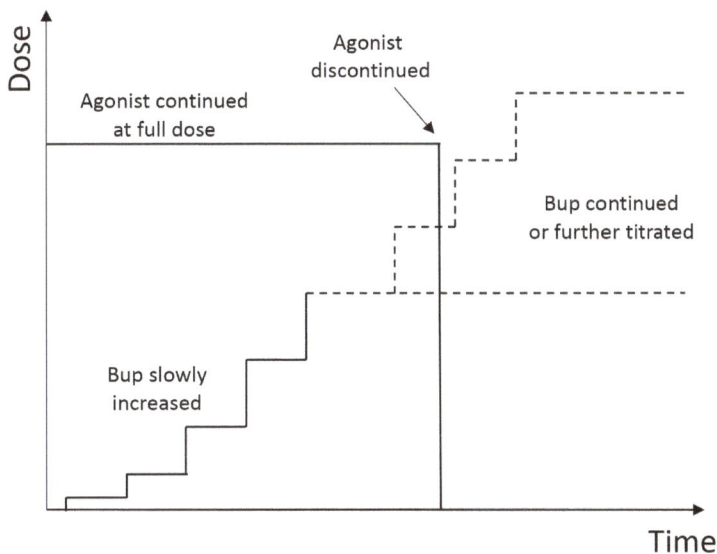

How to Do Microinduction

There is no standard microinduction protocol, at least not yet. You can use either sublingual or transdermal formulations of buprenorphine. The challenge is that it can be hard to procure the very low doses required, since microinduction starts with 0.5 mg or 1 mg doses—a fraction of the 2–8 mg formulations usually available. Films are easier than tablets to divide into small doses since tablets tend to crumble if split into quarters or eighths. Here is a sample protocol, which you should adjust as needed depending on your patient's response:

Day	Buprenorphine Dosage	Opioid Agonist Dosage
1	0.5 mg once	Full dose
2	0.5 mg BID	Full dose
3	1 mg BID	Full dose
4	2 mg BID	Full dose
5	2 mg TID	Full dose
6	2 mg QID	Full dose
7	4 mg TID	Stop
8+	Titrate as usual	

1. Ensure that your patient is currently taking a consistent dose of their current opioid agonist, such as oxycodone, methadone, etc.

2. Start patient on very small doses of buprenorphine using the accompanying chart as a guide. Buprenorphine with naloxone is the standard choice if using sublingual formulations.

3. Have patient stop their current opioid—typically patients can tolerate abruptly stopping the full agonist once they are on 8–12 mg total daily dose of buprenorphine.

How to Use Sublocade and Brixadi

Sublocade and Brixadi are long-acting forms of injectable buprenorphine given once every four or eight weeks for Sublocade and weekly or monthly for Brixadi. The ease of use and flexible dosing of these extended-release formulations make them real game-changers, particularly for patients with adherence challenges. Both products are expensive, though Medicare and many Medicaid programs cover the cost. See "Buprenorphine Extended-Release Injection Monotherapy" fact sheet for additional information.

Sublocade comes as a prefilled syringe in two doses: 100 mg/0.5 mL and 300 mg/1.5 mL. It is given as a subcutaneous intra-abdominal injection. The needle is short but rather thick, so it can hurt going in, though the pain subsides after a few seconds. It forms a small deposit, a little smaller than a grape, that slowly releases medication for up to 18 months.

Patients should be stabilized on sublingual or buccal buprenorphine for at least five days prior to receiving their first injection. The Sublocade dosage depends on how much buprenorphine it took to stabilize symptoms:

SL/Buccal Dose	Sublocade Dose		
	First dose	Second dose (four weeks later)	Maintenance dose
8–18 mg daily	300 mg	100 mg*	100 mg Q4wks or 300 mg Q8wks
20–24 mg daily	300 mg	300 mg	100 mg Q4wks

*If patient is still experiencing craving or withdrawal after initial dose, consider 300 mg as second dose

- Some patients have breakthrough cravings on the 100 mg dose. For these patients, you can give 300 mg every month indefinitely. Anecdotally, this situation is common.
- You can forgo the five-day trial period for patients who have previously tolerated buprenorphine and have an established dose.
- Serum levels peak about 24 hours after injection. Some patients will require one or two doses of sublingual or buccal buprenorphine before the Sublocade takes full effect.
- Shortest duration between doses is 26 days.

Brixadi comes in a range of doses in prefilled syringes (see fact sheet). It is given as a subcutaneous injection into the buttocks, thigh, abdomen, or upper arms (avoid upper arms for first four doses).

Unlike Sublocade, Brixadi can be initiated in patients not already receiving sublingual or buccal buprenorphine, but a 4 mg SL dose is recommended to help determine dosing.

SL/Buccal Dose	Brixadi Weekly Dose	Brixadi Monthly Dose
≤6 mg daily	8 mg	N/A
8–10 mg daily	16 mg	64 mg
12–16 mg daily	24 mg	96 mg
18–24 mg daily	32 mg	128 mg

When transitioning from Brixadi weekly to Brixadi monthly dosing (or vice versa), use the following dosing guide:
- 16 mg weekly: use 64 mg monthly
- 24 mg weekly: use 96 mg monthly
- 32 mg weekly: use 128 mg monthly

Who is eligible:
- Patients with poor adherence to sublingual/buccal buprenorphine
- Patients who travel and may be stuck out of town without medication
- Patients who prefer to minimize pill burden
- Patients in unstable social situations, like being unhoused or leaving incarceration

Tips for administration:
- Needle enters at a 45-degree angle for Sublocade, 90-degree angle for Brixadi
- Give the medication over a minute or so; very fast injections hurt more
- Do not rub the injection area after the injection
- Avoid injecting at the belt line or where a seatbelt will cross

How to Manage and Taper Buprenorphine

Early Treatment

After you have initiated buprenorphine, see patients weekly at first to make sure the dose is right. Increase the dose if they are experiencing cravings—the maximum dose is typically 24 mg daily. Doses can be split if patients are having withdrawal symptoms between doses. Multiple doses per day can be helpful for patients with chronic pain. For most patients, the optimal dose will be 16–24 mg daily. Eventually you can see patients monthly.

Managing Side Effects

- Constipation is the most common side effect. All patients starting buprenorphine should be given docusate/senna, which can be increased up to three tabs BID. Polyethylene glycol, magnesium citrate, and suppositories can be used if docusate/senna is insufficient.
- Some patients have reactions to the naloxone in co-formulated buprenorphine/naloxone. Headache is the most common symptom, but GI distress and anxiety can also be seen. Try switching to buprenorphine monoproduct for these patients.
- Because it's a partial agonist, sedation from buprenorphine alone is uncommon. If patients are reporting sedation, look for other CNS depressants, either prescribed or illicit, such as benzos, muscle relaxants, or alcohol.

Buprenorphine Maintenance vs Tapering

- The best outcomes are with long-term treatment. Overdose risk skyrockets once the medication is stopped. Encourage patients to continue taking the medication.
- If the patient insists on stopping, buprenorphine should be tapered slowly (see "Opioid Withdrawal Management" fact sheet).
  - Proceed in 4 mg increments initially, but slow down toward the end to 1 mg at a time.
  - Decrease dose once every few days to few weeks as tolerated.
  - Films can be cut into small pieces; they are easier to use than tablets for small increments.
  - Adjunctive clonidine can be helpful toward the end of the taper.

If Buprenorphine Doesn't Work

- *Encourage social support.* In conjunction with buprenorphine, ongoing substance use treatment, peer support groups like Alcoholics Anonymous (AA), and sober friends and family can be invaluable in helping patients through the ups and downs of early recovery.
- *Consider methadone.* For some patients, the partial agonism of buprenorphine just isn't enough. Methadone is a good option for patients who continue to experience cravings on 24 mg of buprenorphine.
- *Assess for diversion.* Buprenorphine can be sold on the street. Patients may be insufficiently treated because they are selling rather than taking their medication. Early refills, incorrect pill counts, and urine drug screens negative for buprenorphine can suggest diversion.

How to Manage Methadone

Introduction

Unless you work in a federally funded methadone clinic, known as an opioid treatment program (OTP), you won't be managing methadone long term or making dose adjustments on your own. Treating OUD patients with methadone for more than a few days requires collaboration with an OTP, so if you have a patient who needs methadone, don't hesitate to reach out to one nearby, if one is available. You will also see patients on methadone for other psychiatric needs, so you need to know some details about how OTPs operate and how methadone can interact with other medications. For those initiating methadone in an inpatient setting and referring to OTP for follow-up, see "Managing Opioid Withdrawal in the Inpatient Setting" fact sheet.

Methadone Clinics

- A typical initial dose is 20–30 mg, given as a liquid diluted with juice or artificially colored water. Each patient receives the same volume of liquid regardless of the dose.
- The dose is titrated up by 5–10 mg every few days, to an initial target range of 60–80 mg daily. Doses are increased more gradually after that, and most patients end up doing best on 80–120 mg per day, though some patients may need substantially more.
- Patients are initially seen daily. Patients can earn "take-home" doses after a certain period of stability. Take-home doses typically start at two days at a time, usually over weekends, but can extend for as long as 28 days in some settings.
- If patients will be out of town, they can arrange ahead of time to go to another clinic for "guest dosing."
- Patients should be encouraged to stay on methadone, but if they insist on discontinuing, methadone should be tapered very slowly over several months. Typical rate is no more than 5 mg per week.
- Dose adjustments must be done by the patient's outpatient methadone provider. If the patient is hospitalized, the prescriber must get in touch with the methadone clinic to confirm dosing and collaborate if adjustments are needed.

Managing Side Effects

- Methadone is a full opioid agonist and therefore a powerful CNS depressant. It will have an additive effect when combined with other opioids.
- Methadone prolongs the QT interval. Be careful about combining it with other QT-prolonging agents (like antipsychotics). ECG monitoring is essential when managing methadone for medically ill patients who are hospitalized.
- Exercise great caution when combining with other CNS depressants.

Methadone and Psychiatric Meds

- Steer clear of combining methadone with benzos and z-drugs.
- Methadone is metabolized primarily by CYP3A4 (and 1A2, 2D6 to a lesser amount).
  - Inhibitors (some antivirals in particular) can increase levels and lead to sedation.
  - Inducers (ie, carbamazepine) can decrease levels and cause opioid withdrawal.
- See "Medication Interactions" fact sheet for more information.

Managing Opioid Withdrawal in the Inpatient Setting

Who Is Likely to Experience Withdrawal Symptoms?
- Risk group: Anyone consistently taking opioids for ≥2 weeks.
- Predictors of severe withdrawal: Daily use, high dosage, and use of short-acting opioids.

Common Symptoms of Opioid Withdrawal
- **FLU OPRS** mnemonic:
    - **F**lu-like: Fever, sweating, chills.
    - **L**eg movements: Restlessness, kicking.
    - **U**nwell: General malaise.
    - **O**veractive reflexes: Twitches, spasms.
    - **P**ain: Muscles, stomach, bones.
    - **R**uns: Diarrhea.
    - **S**leep: Insomnia.

Withdrawal Time Course
- Fentanyl: onset 3–12 hours, peak 12–36 hours, duration 5–7 days
- Heroin: onset 8–24 hours, peak 36–72 hours, duration 7–10 days
- Short-acting analgesics (eg, hydrocodone, oxycodone): onset 6–12 hours, peak 12–36 hours, duration 5–7 days
- Long-acting analgesics (eg, morphine): onset 8–24 hours, peak 36–72 hours, duration 7–10 days
- Methadone: onset 1–3 days, peak 4–7 days, duration 2–4 weeks

Severity Measurement
- *Clinical Opiate Withdrawal Scale (COWS)*: Clinician-administered (see page 25).

Management of Withdrawal Symptoms
- Opioid-assisted: Can use either buprenorphine or methadone (though buprenorphine is most common)
    - Buprenorphine
        - Start when patient is in mild/moderate withdrawal (COWS score of 8–12).
        - Prescribe 4 mg SL, then reevaluate your patient after 30–45 minutes to assess withdrawal symptoms and determine if redosing of another 4 mg SL buprenorphine is necessary.
        - Reevaluate your patient after another 30–45 minutes and administer another 4 mg SL buprenorphine if the patient still has a COWS score of 8–12.
        - A total of 8–12 mg SL buprenorphine is usually sufficient to prevent physiologic withdrawal symptoms in the first 24 hours.
        - Titrate the daily dose by 8 mg/day to a maximum of 24 mg daily with the goal of eliminating opioid cravings. Most patients will need 16–24 mg to eliminate cravings completely.
        - Once a maintenance dose is determined, administer it daily, or divided BID or TID.
        - Encourage patients to remain on buprenorphine long term, as they'll otherwise face a high risk of returning to use after discharge. Remember to refer them for outpatient buprenorphine treatment.
    - Methadone
        - Some patients have difficulty tolerating buprenorphine and seem to be prone to experiencing precipitated withdrawal. Consider using methadone for these patients instead.
        - Start with 20–30 mg of methadone as an initial dose. Reassess your patient after two to four hours and administer another 5–10 mg if they are still experiencing withdrawal symptoms.
        - A dose of 40 mg should be sufficient to prevent physiologic withdrawal symptoms in the first 24 hours.
        - Any patient receiving methadone for OUD for more than 72 hours needs to be connected to a federally regulated opioid treatment program (OTP). Contact local programs and ensure that the patient has follow-up if you plan on continuing methadone.
        - Collaborate with the OTP on dosing. Typical titration rates are 5–10 mg every few days with the goal of eliminating cravings. Doses may need to be as high as 120 mg or above.
        - Once the patient is stable, administer the total daily dose once daily.

- Symptom-based treatment—when opioid withdrawal management with buprenorphine or methadone is not available
  - Autonomic symptoms (GI distress, anxiety, sweating, cramping): clonidine 0.1–0.2 mg Qhr; max 0.8 mg/day. Check blood pressure before each dose.
  - Nausea: Ondansetron 4 mg Q4–6hrs; max 16 mg/day.
  - Anxiety: Lorazepam 1 mg Q4–6hrs; max 4 mg/day.
  - Diarrhea: Loperamide 4 mg, then 2 mg after each loose stool; max 16 mg/day.
  - Cramps: Dicyclomine: 10–20 mg Q6hrs.
  - Muscle spasm: Methocarbamol: 750–1500 mg Q8hrs or cyclobenzaprine: 5–10 mg Q6hrs; max 30 mg/day.

How to Discuss and Initiate Extended-Release Naltrexone (Vivitrol)

Introduction

Extended-release naltrexone injection (XR-NTX) is an effective medication for some patients with opioid use disorder (OUD). Oral naltrexone has very weak evidence in OUD, so stick to the injectable form. It works by blocking opioid receptors, which can decrease drug cravings and prevent opioid effects if the patient does use. Because XR-NTX is an opioid blocker, patients must be opioid-free when they receive their first dose; otherwise, they could experience severe withdrawal. The need for drug abstinence before starting XR-NTX is its biggest drawback.

How to Discuss XR-NTX With Patients

Proper adherence is important to emphasize for long-acting injectables; the long interval between doses can make it easy for some patients to forget about follow-up. Patients also must understand that naltrexone is an opioid blocker and therefore won't ease withdrawal symptoms like buprenorphine or methadone. Finally, patients need to understand that it is crucial to be opioid-free before getting the first dose (and for the duration of treatment), or a very uncomfortable and drawn-out precipitated withdrawal could result.

Step 1: Ensure Your Patient Is Opioid-Free

In order to avoid precipitated withdrawal, patients need to have all opioids out of their system before their first dose. That usually starts with a medically supervised management of withdrawal symptoms. Since they can't have any opioids on board, that means no buprenorphine or methadone; withdrawal has to be managed utilizing a symptom-triggered protocol with clonidine and other symptomatic agents (see "Opioid Withdrawal: Time Course and Symptoms" fact sheet). They will need to be abstinent from short-acting opioids (eg, morphine, oxycodone, heroin) for seven to 10 days and long-acting opioids (eg, methadone, buprenorphine, street fentanyl) for 10–14 days before XR-NTX is given.

Step 2: Screen to Ensure the Patient Is Ready

Get a rapid urine drug screen and make sure that it is negative for opioids. Be sure the screen includes fentanyl and buprenorphine, as not all do. If the screen is positive, don't give XR-NTX. Repeat the screen every 24 hours until it is negative. Once negative, you can give XR-NTX. Some patients may have an incentive to begin treatment as soon as possible (for example, to satisfy treatment program requirements or a court mandate). Others might be embarrassed that they returned to use during a period of trying to maintain sobriety. So if the urine tox turns negative earlier than expected, or you are suspicious about the results, consider a naloxone challenge test by administering a small dose of naloxone (0.2 mg IV or 0.8 mg SC). Any withdrawal symptoms caused by naloxone will be short-lived and will tell you that the patient isn't ready for XR-NTX. If they don't have any withdrawal, they can get XR-NTX.

Step 3: Give XR-NTX as a Single Gluteal Injection

Each injection is 380 mg and comes as a powder that needs to be reconstituted with saline before administration. The reconstituted medication is 4 mL of a viscous liquid that is given as a deep IM gluteal injection every four weeks. Use a 1.5-inch needle for thin patients and a 2-inch needle for larger patients. It's normal to be sore for a few days at the injection site—ice and OTC analgesics can help.

Step 4: Repeat Injection Every Four Weeks

XR-NTX is designed to be given every 28 days, though the effect can wear off a little early in some patients. If this is the case, they can get the medication every three weeks.

Extended-Release Naltrexone Cheat Sheet

1. Patients must be abstinent from opioids for seven to 14 days before first dose
2. Ensure all opioids are out of their system with a urine tox or naloxone challenge
3. Warn patients about a few days of soreness at the injection site
4. Repeat doses every three to four weeks

Medication Interactions

Introduction

Opioid use disorder (OUD) is highly comorbid with medical illness and other psychiatric conditions. Most of your patients on medications for OUD (MOUD) will also be taking other medications (Du CX et al, *Fam Pract* 2022;39(2): 234–240). MOUDs generally play well with other medications, but there are some important interactions to be aware of. Here is a summary of some important med-med interactions to be wary of when prescribing MOUDs.

Central Nervous System (CNS) Depression

The CNS depressant effects of buprenorphine and methadone can be compounded when combined with other sedating medications. Two classes of commonly prescribed medications warrant particular caution (but also be careful with alcohol, barbiturates, and other CNS depressants):

- *Benzodiazepines:* These can have powerful CNS depressant effects, including respiratory suppression, which are additive with those of opioids. Benzo prescriptions are associated with an increased risk of opioid overdose death (Park T et al, *Addiction* 2020;115(5):924–932) and generally should be used only with great caution in those taking an MOUD.

- *Gabapentinoids:* Gabapentin and pregabalin are not particularly dangerous on their own but have increasingly been implicated in opioid overdose deaths in postmortem studies (Mattson CL et al, *Morb Mortal Wkly Rep* 2022;71(19):664–666). While they are almost certainly safer to prescribe than benzos, we recommend caution when combining them with buprenorphine or methadone, especially for those continuing to use illicit opioids.

P450 Interactions

Buprenorphine and methadone are primarily metabolized by CYP3A4, with smaller contributions from other P450 enzyme subsystems. The key is to look out for major inducers and inhibitors, which can affect serum levels. Here are the big ones to know:

- *Inducers:* These lower the serum concentration of buprenorphine and methadone, meaning patients may require higher than expected doses or a dose adjustment when the offending agent is discontinued. If the patient is already on an MOUD and an inducer is started, they may have breakthrough opioid cravings or withdrawal symptoms.
  - Carbamazepine
  - Phenobarbital
  - Phenytoin
  - Rifampin
  - St. John's wort

- *Inhibitors:* These raise the serum concentration of buprenorphine and methadone, meaning patients may require less medication than usual. If the patient is already on an MOUD and an inhibitor is started, they may get sedated. Many antifungals, many antivirals, and some antibacterial agents are strong CYP3A4 inhibitors. As this list is not comprehensive, we recommend utilizing a medication interaction checker such as Micromedex when a new medication is started.
  - Clarithromycin, erythromycin
  - Diltiazem, verapamil
  - Fluvoxamine
  - Grapefruit juice
  - Nefazodone: atypical antidepressant
  - Azole antifungals (itraconazole, fluconazole, ketoconazole, etc)
  - Many antiretroviral medications (atazanavir, delavirdine, indinavir, ritonavir, etc)

Cardiac Issues

Methadone is a well-known QT-prolonging medication. Buprenorphine can prolong the QT interval as well, though to a lesser extent. Perhaps surprisingly, injectable naltrexone is associated with prolonged QT and cardiac arrhythmias as well (Raji MA et al, *Am J Med* 2022;135(7):864–870). Use caution when prescribing an MOUD to patients who have preexisting heart disease or are receiving other QT-prolonging agents such as:

- Many antiarrhythmics (always double-check these)
- Citalopram and escitalopram
- Donepezil
- Pimozide
- IV haloperidol
- IV ondansetron
- Low-potency first-generation antipsychotics
- Azole antifungals (see above)
- Fluoroquinolones (end in "-floxacin": levofloxacin, ciprofloxacin, etc)
- Macrolides (end in "-mycin": erythromycin, clarithromycin, etc)
- VMAT2 inhibitors

Pain Management for Patients With Opioid Use Disorder

Introduction

Pain and opioid use disorder (OUD) are tightly intertwined and highly comorbid. OUD arises in some patients who receive opioids as treatment for acute or chronic pain. Opioid misuse can provide potent analgesia, and opioid withdrawal can exacerbate pain. Treating chronic pain in patients with OUD is a challenge, but keeping the following principles in mind can be helpful.

Optimize Non-Opioid Analgesia

There are many classes of non-opioid analgesics, many of which can be combined to augment one another. Optimal treatment usually entails taking medications on a standing basis, and not just as needed. The doses listed are typical treatment ranges, though many of these medications require a titration at the beginning and a taper if they are discontinued. Consider liver and kidney function when choosing a medication and determining dose. Here are some to consider:

- *Acetaminophen:* up to 3000 mg daily in divided doses
- *NSAIDs:* ibuprofen (400–800 mg TID), naproxen (500 mg BID), meloxicam (5–10 mg daily)
- *SNRIs:* duloxetine (30–60 mg daily), venlafaxine (75–225 mg daily)
- *Tricyclics:* nortriptyline (25–75 mg QHS), amitriptyline (25–125 mg QHS)
- *Gabapentinoids:* gabapentin (300–1200 mg TID), pregabalin (150–300 mg BID)
- *Muscle relaxants* (for short-term use): cyclobenzaprine (5–10 mg TID), methocarbamol (up to 4.5 g daily in divided doses)
- *Topicals:* lidocaine cream, lidocaine patches, diclofenac gel, capsaicin cream, menthol

Don't Overlook Non-Pharmacological Interventions

Encourage patients to engage in non-pharmacological interventions that are both behavioral and cognitive, such as:

- Physical therapy
- Mindfulness
- Regular exercise
- Massage therapy
- Cognitive behavioral therapy for pain

Consider Injection Treatments

Consultation with a physiatrist, orthopedist, or neurologist can determine if certain percutaneous procedures may be beneficial. Some commonly performed interventions include:

- Local anesthetic
- Glucocorticoid injection
- Trigger-point injection
- Botox injection
- Radiofrequency ablation

Prescribe Buprenorphine

Though commonly used as a treatment for OUD, buprenorphine was in fact originally developed as an analgesic. Low-dose forms of buprenorphine (transdermal and buccal formulations) are approved for pain treatment but are insufficient for patients with OUD. Nonetheless, buprenorphine at typical OUD treatment doses, namely 16–24 mg, can be effective for pain. Consider dividing doses to multiple times a day, which provides better round-the-clock pain control compared to once-a-day dosing.

Prescribe Methadone

Like buprenorphine, methadone can provide significant pain control while treating OUD at the same time. Patients on methadone for OUD and pain treatment will still need to obtain medication through a federally regulated opioid treatment program and may require doses on the high end of the usual range (ie, >120 mg daily).

Consult With a Pain Specialist

If pain is still inadequately controlled despite your best efforts, consider consulting a pain specialist, who may have more expertise in treating comorbid OUD and chronic pain.

How to Educate Your Patients About Overdose Prevention

Introduction

Drug overdose deaths, the vast majority of which involve opioids, continue to rise in the US. Health care providers should be able to identify patients at particularly high risk for overdose, know how to mitigate risk using harm reduction strategies, and educate patients to recognize and quickly treat overdose. (See "Opioid Overdose Overview Fact Sheet for Patients.")

Risk Factors for Overdose

Certain patient characteristics are associated with a particularly elevated risk of overdose; monitor these patients as closely as possible. Some risk factors are "static" and do not change, including:

- Prior history of overdose
- History of high dose or quantity of use
- Chronic medical illnesses that impact lung, liver, or kidney function

Other risk factors, called "dynamic," are changeable. Discuss these dynamic factors with your patients, determine which ones pose the most risk, and counsel them on harm reduction strategies that can lower the risk of fatal overdose:

Dynamic Overdose Risk Factor	Harm Reduction Strategy
Loss of opioid tolerance	• Use less after a period of abstinence, even a few days • Start with a tester dose • Use intranasally over intravenously
Mixing drugs	• Use one drug at a time • If mixing, use opioid first
High potency	• Keep a consistent dealer • Talk to others who have used from same batch • If a new drug source, start with a small tester dose • Test each new batch of drugs for fentanyl using fentanyl test strips
Using alone	• Don't use alone • Tell people if you are going to use alone • Call the Never Use Alone hotline: (877) 696-1996

How to Recognize an Opioid Overdose

Patients do not give naloxone to themselves when they are overdosing! It is essential that your patients know how to recognize an overdose and know how to respond. That way, they can teach their friends and family what to look out for and what to do in case they overdose. Signs of overdose include:

- Slow or absent breathing
- Signs of obstructed airway (wheezing, snoring, gurgling)
- Not responsive to sternal rub
- Pinpoint pupils
- Cold or clammy skin
- Blue or grayish coloration of lips, fingernails, or skin
- Thready or weak pulse

Overdose Response

Teach your patients the following steps to follow in case an overdose is suspected. They can pass this information along to friends and family, and also tell them where they keep their naloxone.

1. *Assess for signs of overdose:* Attempt to arouse patient with sternal rub. If that is not effective, move on to the next step.
2. *Call 911:* Say "Someone is unresponsive and not breathing." Give clear address and location.
3. *Administer naloxone or nalmefene:* If the patient does not respond to a single dose in the first two or three minutes, administer another dose into the other nostril. Doses can be repeated every two to three minutes until arrival of EMS.
4. *Support ABCs:* Assess for presence of pulse and respirations.
   - If no pulse or respirations, deliver CPR.
   - If pulse is present but no respirations, deliver rescue breathing.
   - Whenever the patient is left on their own, place in the rescue position in order to avoid aspiration. The patient should be on their side, hand under head, supported with elbow and knee.
5. *Monitor response:* Provide supportive care until EMS arrives. If the patient awakens, ensure that they do not use more opioids. Never leave the patient alone.

Medication Fact Sheets

BUPRENORPHINE EXTENDED-RELEASE INJECTION MONOTHERAPY (Brixadi, Sublocade) Fact Sheet

Bottom Line:
Extended-release injectable formulations of buprenorphine allow patients to receive doses weekly, monthly, or every eight weeks for patients maintained on a low dose—which improves medication adherence. Brixadi has the advantage over Sublocade due to its more flexible dosing options.

FDA Indications:
Opioid use disorder (maintenance).

Dosage Forms:
- **Monthly injection (Sublocade):** 100 mg/0.5 mL, 300 mg/1.5 mL prefilled syringes.
- **Weekly or monthly injection (Brixadi):** 8 mg, 16 mg, 24 mg, 32 mg (weekly) and 64 mg, 96 mg, 128 mg (monthly) prefilled syringes.

Dosage Guidance:
- After patient is stabilized on sublingual (SL) buprenorphine for seven days:
  - Sublocade:
    - Injections are given subcutaneously in the abdomen.
    - For patients maintained on 8–18 mg: Start with 300 mg then 100 mg monthly or 300 mg Q8wks.
    - For patients maintained on 20–24 mg: Start with 300 mg monthly for two months, then give 100 mg monthly maintenance doses.
    - Patients commonly have opioid cravings or withdrawal symptoms when dropping down to the 100 mg dose. For these patients, you can give 300 mg every month.
    - Doses may be given early if clinically indicated, though no closer than 26 days apart.
  - Brixadi:
    - Injections are given subcutaneously in the buttocks, thigh, abdomen, or upper arms (upper arm should be avoided for first four doses).
    - Rotate administration sites for weekly injections and avoid administering into same site for at least eight weeks. No site rotation needed for monthly injections.
    - For patients maintained on ≤6 mg: Give 8 mg weekly.
    - For patients maintained on 8–10 mg: Give 16 mg weekly or 64 mg monthly.
    - For patients maintained on 12–16 mg: Give 24 mg weekly or 96 mg monthly.
    - For patients maintained on 18–24 mg: Give 32 mg weekly or 128 mg monthly.

Monitoring: Baseline and monthly LFTs.

Cost: $$$$

Side Effects:
- Most common: Injection site itching and pain, constipation, headache, insomnia, nausea, anxiety.
- Serious but rare: Hepatitis reported rarely, ranging from transient, asymptomatic transaminase elevations to hepatic failure; in many cases, patients had preexisting hepatic dysfunction. Respiratory depression and orthostatic hypotension possible.
- Boxed warning emphasizes the risk of administering the drug intravenously rather than the intended subcutaneous route. Their gel formulations could cause occlusion, local tissue damage, or thrombotic events if injected intravenously, potentially causing severe harm or death.

Mechanism, Pharmacokinetics, and Drug Interactions:
- Partial opioid agonist (delta and mu receptors) and antagonist (kappa receptors).
- Metabolized primarily through CYP3A4; t ½: 24–48 hours.
- Avoid concomitant use with opioid analgesics (diminished pain control). Additive effects with CNS depressants. CYP3A4 inhibitors and inducers may affect levels of buprenorphine.

Clinical Pearls:

- Schedule III controlled substance. Prescribing buprenorphine for OUD no longer requires having a special "X-license."
- Extended-release injectable formulations are only available through a REMS program.
- Of the two formulations, Brixadi offers more flexibility in terms of dosing and injection sites.
- If needed in first week, can give an additional 8 mg weekly injection of Brixadi (at least 24 hours after previous injection). Dose adjustments can be made weekly with a maximum weekly dose of 32 mg.
- Brixadi can be switched from weekly to monthly or vice versa based on the following equivalencies: 16 mg weekly = 64 mg monthly, 24 mg weekly = 96 mg monthly, 32 mg weekly = 128 mg monthly.
- Brixadi weekly can be initiated in patients not currently receiving SL buprenorphine, but a 4 mg SL test dose is recommended to help determine appropriate dose.

Fun Fact:

- The development of long-lasting buprenorphine injections represents a milestone in "depot technology," where the medication is stored and gradually released in the body, reducing the need for daily dosing and potentially improving treatment outcomes.

BUPRENORPHINE MONOTHERAPY (Subutex, others) Fact Sheet [G]

Bottom Line:

Buprenorphine (Subutex, available now only as generic) is the active ingredient in Suboxone (buprenorphine/naloxone) and is responsible for the effectiveness of the combination medication in opioid use disorder (OUD). In the past, buprenorphine alone was preferred for the initial (induction) phase of treatment, while Suboxone was preferred for maintenance treatment (unsupervised administration). Currently, the combination is favored for both induction and maintenance as it, at least theoretically, decreases misuse and diversion.

FDA Indications:

OUD: induction, maintenance; moderate to severe pain (Belbuca, Buprenex, Butrans).

Dosage Forms:

- **SL tablets (Subutex, [G]):** 2 mg, 8 mg (scored).
- **Buccal film (Belbuca, [G]):** 75 mcg, 150 mcg, 300 mcg, 450 mcg, 600 mcg, 750 mcg, 900 mcg (used for pain).
- **Transdermal patch (Butrans):** 5 mcg/hr, 7.5 mcg/hr, 10 mcg/hr, 15 mcg/hr, 20 mcg/hr (used for pain).
- **Short-acting injection (Buprenex, [G]):** 0.3 mg/mL (used for pain).
- **Extended-release injection:** For OUD; see "Buprenorphine Extended-Release Injection Monotherapy" fact sheet.

Dosage Guidance for OUD:

- Induction procedure (SL tablets):
  - Begin when opioid withdrawal reaches moderate severity; otherwise, you may trigger withdrawal symptoms.
  - Start 4–8 mg SL day 1; increase up to 16 mg on day 2; then up to 24 mg on day 3. Some patients may need up to 12 mg in first 24 hours. Typical maintenance dose is 8–24 mg SL QD, though best evidence is for 16–24 mg; max 32 mg/day.
  - See separate fact sheets for more information about induction procedures.

Monitoring: No routine monitoring recommended unless clinical picture warrants.

Cost: SL: $$

Side Effects:

- Most common: Constipation, headache, insomnia, nausea, anxiety.
- Serious but rare: Hepatitis reported rarely, ranging from transient, asymptomatic transaminase elevations to hepatic failure; in many cases, patients had preexisting hepatic dysfunction. QT prolongation, particularly with higher doses of transdermal patch. Rare cases of dental problems including tooth decay, cavities, and infections; recommend swishing with water after dose completely dissolved and good dental care.

Mechanism, Pharmacokinetics, and Drug Interactions:

- Partial opioid agonist (delta and mu receptors) and antagonist (kappa receptors).
- Metabolized primarily through CYP3A4; t ½: 24–48 hours.
- Avoid concomitant use with opioid analgesics (diminished pain control). Additive effects with CNS depressants. CYP3A4 inhibitors and inducers may affect levels of buprenorphine.

Clinical Pearls:

- Schedule III controlled substance. Prescribing buprenorphine for OUD no longer requires having a special "X-license."
- Though buprenorphine/naloxone products are recommended for maintenance treatment, buprenorphine monoproduct can be used during pregnancy and for the handful of patients who may have adverse effects to the small amount of naloxone absorbed sublingually from the combination product (headache, anxiety, GI distress, palpitations).
- Patients with moderate to severe OUD and who have been stabilized with SL or buccal buprenorphine 8–24 mg for >7 days may convert to monthly or weekly subcutaneous injections.

Fun Fact:

The subcutaneous implant formulation of buprenorphine (Probuphine) was discontinued. Its use was severely limited as it was invasive, expensive, and an option only for patients stable on ≤8 mg/day of SL buprenorphine. Other implants currently in development include medications for schizophrenia, breast cancer, photosensitivity, and Parkinson's disease.

BUPRENORPHINE/NALOXONE (Bunavail, Suboxone, Zubsolv) Fact Sheet [G]

Bottom Line:

Buprenorphine/naloxone is the definitive partial agonist treatment for opioid use disorder (OUD). The combination product is preferred over buprenorphine alone for maintenance because it is the most widely available formulation and the addition of naloxone might lower its potential for misuse. The sublingual film formulation is priced a little higher than the sublingual tablets yet provides very little (if any) clinically meaningful benefit; generic tablets should be favored as a cost-saving measure.

FDA Indications:

OUD (induction and maintenance).

Dosage Forms:

- **SL tablets (G):** 2/0.5 mg, 8/2 mg (scored).
- **SL film strips (Suboxone, [G]):** 2/0.5 mg, 4/1 mg, 8/2 mg, 12/3 mg.
- **SL tablets (Zubsolv):** 0.7/0.18 mg, 1.4/0.36 mg, 2.9/0.71 mg, 5.7/1.4 mg, 8.6/2.1 mg, 11.4/2.9 mg.
- **Buccal film (Bunavail):** 2.1/0.3 mg, 4.2/0.7 mg, 6.3/1 mg.

Dosage Guidance:

- Induction procedure:
    - Begin when opioid withdrawal reaches moderate severity; otherwise you may trigger more severe withdrawal symptoms.
    - Start 4–8 mg SL day 1; increase up to 16 mg on day 2; then up to 24 mg on day 3. Some patients may need up to 12 mg in first 24 hours.
- Maintenance treatment: Give combination product (Suboxone or [G]) daily in the equivalent buprenorphine dose on last day of induction; adjust dose in increments between 2 mg and 8 mg to a level that suppresses opioid cravings (usually 8–24 mg/day); best evidence is for 16–24 mg/day; max 32 mg/day.
- Some patients prefer taking smaller doses multiple times per day; can be a useful strategy for chronic pain patients.
- Zubsolv 5.7/1.4 mg SL tablet provides equivalent buprenorphine to Suboxone 8/2 mg SL tablet.
- Bunavail 4.2/0.7 mg buccal film provides equivalent buprenorphine to Suboxone 8/2 mg SL tablet.

Monitoring: No routine monitoring recommended unless clinical picture warrants.

Cost: SL tablet, film, Bunavail: $–$$ depending on dose; Zubsolv: $$$

Side Effects:

- Most common: Constipation, headache, vomiting, sweating.
- Serious but rare: Hepatitis reported rarely, ranging from transient, asymptomatic transaminase elevations to hepatic failure; in many cases, patients had preexisting hepatic dysfunction. Rare cases of dental problems including tooth decay, cavities, and infections; recommend swishing with water after dose completely dissolved and good dental care.

Mechanism, Pharmacokinetics, and Drug Interactions:

- Buprenorphine: Partial opioid agonist (delta and mu receptors) and antagonist (kappa receptors); naloxone: Opioid antagonist (mu receptor).
- Metabolized primarily through CYP3A4; t ½: 24–48 hours (naloxone: 2–12 hours).
- Avoid concomitant use with opiate analgesics (diminished pain control). Additive effects with CNS depressants. CYP3A4 inhibitors and inducers may affect levels of buprenorphine.

Clinical Pearls:

- Schedule III controlled substance. Prescribing buprenorphine for OUD no longer requires having a special "X-license."
- Naloxone is an opioid antagonist that is active only when injected; it is added to buprenorphine in order to reduce misuse via intravenous injection of a dissolved tablet.
- The SL film formulation's manufacturer claims it dissolves faster and tastes better than SL tablets. Actually, it is more likely a way for the manufacturer to switch users to a "new" product (with patent protection until 2025) rather than lose patients to generics. There is no evidence to suggest that there is any clinical benefit.

- SL film should be placed at base of tongue to the side of midline; this allows patient to use two tablets or films at the same time if dose dictates.
- Zubsolv and Bunavail formulations have better bioavailability, hence the dose equivalencies noted above.
- Prescribers should be aware of the risk for diversion and sale of buprenorphine films and tablets. Buprenorphine is bought and sold on the streets typically to combat cravings and withdrawal symptoms.

Fun Fact:

The manufacturer of Suboxone, Reckitt Benckiser, generates most of its revenue from selling home and personal care products like Lysol cleaners and Durex condoms.

LOFEXIDINE (Lucemyra) Fact Sheet

Bottom Line:
Lofexidine is an alpha-2 agonist (similar to clonidine and guanfacine) that is used to reduce the intensity of opioid withdrawal symptoms. It effectively blunts some of the most distressing symptoms such as anxiety and tachycardia. It is generally not effective for pain symptoms such as generalized achiness and headache, so it should be used with an analgesic like ibuprofen or acetaminophen. Data indicate that lofexidine is similarly effective to clonidine for management of opioid withdrawal but with a marginally better side effect profile (Kuszmaul AK et al, *J Am Pharm Assoc* 2020;60(1):145–152). However, given its much higher price tag, we recommend you stick to clonidine.

FDA Indications:
Opioid withdrawal.

Dosage Forms:
Tablets: 0.18 mg.

Dosage Guidance:
- Start three 0.18 mg tablets QID at five- to six-hour intervals during peak withdrawal symptoms (typically the first five to seven days after last use of opioid). Withdrawal symptoms should be used clinically to guide gradual dose reduction.
- Maximum daily dose is 2.88 mg (16 tablets), and no single dose should exceed 0.72 mg (four tablets).
- Discontinue gradually by reducing in increments of one tablet per dose every one to two days. Taper typically should take two to four days, and should be no more than 14 days.

Monitoring: Monitor blood pressure and pulse. Monitor ECG in patients with congestive heart failure, bradyarrhythmia, or risk for QT prolongation.

Cost: $$$$

Side Effects:
- Most common: Orthostatic hypotension, bradycardia, dizziness, somnolence, sedation, dry mouth.
- Serious but rare: Syncope, QT interval prolongation.

Mechanism, Pharmacokinetics, and Drug Interactions:
- Alpha-2 receptor agonist.
- Metabolized primarily by CYP2D6; t ½: 11–12 hours.
- Caution when used with CYP2D6 inhibitors (such as paroxetine) or in poor 2D6 metabolizers as there may be an increased risk for hypotension. Caution with other agents that may increase QT interval (eg, methadone). Caution when used with CNS depressants (additive CNS depression).

Clinical Pearls:
- Analog of clonidine, another alpha-2 agonist, available since 1992 in the UK.
- Has been approved for use in Europe since the 1990s, but was not approved by the FDA until 2018. Approval was based on two randomized, double-blind, placebo-controlled clinical trials of 866 adults with opioid dependence; lofexidine lessened severity of withdrawal symptoms more than placebo.
- Decide on how rapidly to taper the dose by using a symptom-triggered assessment such as the Clinical Opiate Withdrawal Scale (see the "COWS" fact sheet for more details).
- Lower the dose if symptomatic hypotension or bradycardia occurs, and in patients with impaired hepatic or renal function.
- Some patients may experience markedly increased blood pressure if the lofexidine dose is lowered or discontinued too quickly. For these patients with rebound hypertension, consider slowing down the taper or temporarily treating with another antihypertensive agent.
- Has been studied for alcohol withdrawal but was not found to be effective.

Fun Fact:
Case reports support its use for hot flashes associated with menopause.

METHADONE (Methadose) Fact Sheet [G]

Bottom Line:

Methadone is a long-acting opioid agonist that is one of the mainstays of opioid use disorder (OUD) treatment, along with buprenorphine. Compared to patients not in treatment, those receiving methadone have lower all-cause mortality, rates of transmissible diseases, criminal convictions, suicide, and even cancer. Methadone for OUD must come from a federally regulated opioid treatment program (OTP), or "methadone clinic." Patients start out by going to the clinic daily, which can be an inconvenience. Disadvantages include the potential for diversion and the possible accumulation of doses due to its long half-life.

FDA Indications:

Opioid dependence; severe pain.

Dosage Forms:

- **Tablets (G):** 5 mg, 10 mg, 40 mg (scored).
- **Oral solution (G):** 10 mg/5 mL, 5 mg/5 mL.
- **Oral concentrate (G):** 10 mg/mL.

Dosage Guidance:

Start 15–30 mg single dose; then 5–10 mg every two to four hours until cessation of withdrawal symptoms; max 40 mg on day 1. Maintenance treatment: Increase daily dose by 5–10 mg every two to three days until the patient is no longer experiencing opioid cravings; 80–120 mg per day is a common maintenance dose for opioid dependence.

Monitoring: ECG if cardiac disease.

Cost: $

Side Effects:

- Most common: Constipation, dizziness, sedation, nausea, sweating.
- Serious but rare: May prolong the QT interval and increase risk for torsades de pointes; caution in patients at risk for QT prolongation, especially with doses >100 mg/day. Severe respiratory depression may occur; use extreme caution during initiation, titration, and conversion from other opioids to methadone. Respiratory depressant effects occur later and persist longer than analgesic effects, possibly contributing to cases of overdose.

Mechanism, Pharmacokinetics, and Drug Interactions:

- Opioid agonist.
- Metabolized primarily through CYP2B6, 2C19, and 3A4 (major); inhibits CYP2D6; t ½: 8–59 hours.
- High potential for interactions. Avoid concomitant use with other potent sedatives or respiratory depressants. Use with caution in patients on medications that are metabolized by CYP2D6, inhibit CYP3A4, prolong the QT interval, or promote electrolyte depletion.

Clinical Pearls:

- Schedule II controlled substance; distribution of 40 mg tablets restricted to authorized opioid addiction treatment facilities.
- Currently, may only be dispensed according to the Substance Abuse and Mental Health Services Administration's (SAMHSA) Center for Substance Abuse Treatment (CSAT) guidelines. Regulations vary by area; consult regulatory agencies and/or methadone treatment facilities. Advocacy efforts to expand methadone treatment beyond federally regulated opioid treatment programs have escalated, particularly after relaxed flexibilities during COVID-19 showed positive outcomes.
- Methadone accumulates with repeated doses; dose may need reduction after three to five days to prevent CNS depressant effects.

Fun Fact:

A persistent but untrue urban legend claims the name "Dolophine" was coined in tribute to Adolf Hitler by its German creators. The name was in fact created after the war by the American branch of Eli Lilly, and the pejorative term "adolphine" (never an actual name of the drug) didn't appear in the US until the early 1970s.

NALMEFENE (Opvee) Fact Sheet [G]

Bottom Line:

Nalmefene is an opioid antagonist that has high affinity for opioid receptors and is more potent and longer acting than naloxone. Whether we need this or the newer nasal spray version remains up for debate. Nalmefene is likely not required for most patients; stick with naloxone (now available over the counter) for opioid overdose.

FDA Indications:

Emergency treatment of known or suspected opioid overdose (ages 12 and up).

Dosage Forms:
- **Intranasal (Opvee):** 2.7 mg/0.1 mL.
- **Injectable (G):** 2 mg/2 mL.

Dosage Guidance:
- Intranasal: Bystander to spray in one nostril; may repeat into other nostril with additional doses every two to five minutes if no or minimal response and until emergency response arrives. The drug is absorbed automatically into the nasal mucosa, which is why it is effective in patients who are unconscious and cannot sniff it.
- Injection: 0.5 mg/70 kg/dose IV/IM/SC ×1; may give additional 1 mg/70 kg/dose after two to five minutes. Max 1.5 mg/70 kg total dose. If known or suspected opioid dependence, start with 0.1 mg/70 kg/dose test dose instead; if no withdrawal, follow recommended dosing.

Monitoring: No routine monitoring recommended unless clinical picture warrants.

Cost: Intranasal: $$$

Side Effects:
- Most common: Symptoms of opioid withdrawal, including body aches, fever, sweating, runny nose, sneezing, piloerection, yawning, weakness, shivering or trembling, nervousness, restlessness or irritability, diarrhea, nausea or vomiting, abdominal cramps, increased blood pressure, and tachycardia.

Mechanism, Pharmacokinetics, and Drug Interactions:
- Opioid antagonist.
- Metabolized primarily in the liver (non-CYP450); t ½: 11 hours.

Clinical Pearls:
- First approved in 1995 as an injectable called Revex, nalmefene was discontinued around 2008 due to low sales. A generic version of the injectable was approved in February 2022 and a nasal spray formulation in 2023 to target the shift to fentanyl and other synthetic opioids now responsible for two-thirds of overdose deaths.
- Harm reduction advocates have argued that higher-potency or longer-lasting opioid antagonists are not necessary and could even seem punitive due to the possibility of a more severe and prolonged precipitated withdrawal (up to six hours vs 30–40 minutes with naloxone).
- Available only with a prescription; by comparison, naloxone is now available over the counter.
- Because treatment of overdose with an intranasal opioid antagonist must be performed by someone other than the patient, instruct prescription recipients to inform those around them that they have nalmefene rescue and ensure that those people have been instructed in recognizing overdose symptoms and administering the medication.
- Overdose symptoms (CNS depression and respiratory depression) may return after initial improvement, or patients may require additional support due to precipitated withdrawal symptoms. Therefore, patients should continue to be monitored and should receive medical attention after emergency dose(s) provided.

Fun Fact:

Several studies have shown limited benefits of nalmefene in reducing alcohol consumption, which is not surprising given its similar mechanism of action to naltrexone.

NALOXONE (Kloxxado, Narcan Nasal Spray, RiVive, Zimhi) Fact Sheet [G]

Bottom Line:

Naloxone is an opioid antagonist that is used to rapidly reverse opioid overdose. It's important to recommend having this life-saving treatment on hand to all your patients with opioid use disorder. We recommend the generic, and now over-the-counter, nasal formulations.

FDA Indications:

Emergency treatment of known or suspected opioid overdose.

Dosage Forms:

- **Intranasal (Narcan Nasal Spray, RiVive, [G]):** 3 mg/0.1 mL, 4 mg/0.1 mL.
- **Intranasal (Kloxxado):** 8 mg/0.1 mL.
- **Injectable prefilled syringe (Zimhi):** 5 mg/0.5 mL.
- **Auto-injector (G):** 10 mg.

Dosage Guidance:

Intranasal: Bystander to spray single dose (3, 4, or 8 mg) in one nostril; may repeat into other nostril with additional doses every two to three minutes if no or minimal response until patient responsive or emergency response arrives. The drug is absorbed automatically into the nasal mucosa, which is why it is effective in patients who are unconscious and cannot sniff it.

Monitoring: No routine monitoring recommended unless clinical picture warrants. Any person revived from an opioid overdose with naloxone should be evaluated in an emergency room.

Cost: Intranasal (generic): $; Kloxxado, Zimhi: $$$

Side Effects:

Most common: Symptoms of opioid withdrawal, including body aches, sweating, runny nose, sneezing, piloerection, yawning, weakness, shivering or trembling, nervousness, restlessness or irritability, diarrhea, nausea or vomiting, abdominal cramps, increased blood pressure, and tachycardia.

Mechanism, Pharmacokinetics, and Drug Interactions:

- Opioid antagonist.
- Metabolized primarily by conjugation (non-P450) in the liver; t ½: 1.36 hours.

Clinical Pearls:

- Because treatment of overdose with this opioid antagonist must be performed by someone other than the patient, instruct recipients to inform those around them that they have naloxone rescue and ensure that those people have been instructed in recognizing overdose symptoms and administering the medication.
- Evzio auto-injector offered a novel device with voice instructions but was very expensive; it has been discontinued by the manufacturer and is no longer available. Zimhi is a new injectable (SC/IM) prefilled syringe for layperson use but comes in a much higher 5 mg dose and delivers nearly five-fold higher peak serum concentrations, which could result in very severe precipitated withdrawal symptoms.
- Like Zimhi, Kloxxado is a higher-dose formulation that was developed to combat the presumed need for repeated doses of naloxone after overdose with higher-potency opioids such as fentanyl. Whether multiple doses are required has been controversial, and use of this high-dose antagonist could result in severe precipitated withdrawal. Kloxxado is likely overkill for most patients—stick to the 4 mg intranasal formulation, which has a proven track record and is less expensive.
- Most opioids have a longer duration of action than naloxone, so it's likely that overdose symptoms (CNS depression and respiratory depression) will return after initial improvement. Therefore, patients should continue to be monitored and should receive medical attention after emergency dose(s) provided.
- Intranasal forms of naloxone rescue administration, if broadly distributed to those at risk, could make overdose rescue a more acceptable and widespread practice. Recently, it's become available over the counter.
- Check out the Prescribe to Prevent website (www.prescribetoprevent.org) for prescriber resources such as webinars, toolkits, patient education materials, and medical-legal resources.

Fun Fact:

The new ultra-high-dose (10 mg) auto-injector formulation is specifically indicated for use by military personnel and chemical incident responders for potential exposure to "ultra-potent weaponized opioids."

NALTREXONE (ReVia, Vivitrol) Fact Sheet [G]

Bottom Line:

Naltrexone, an opioid antagonist, is the first-line medication for alcohol use disorder—though it is also approved for opioid use disorder (OUD). By reducing the endorphin-mediated euphoria of drinking, it helps people moderate, preventing that first drink from leading to several more. Avoid naltrexone in patients with hepatic impairment or those taking opioid-based pain medications. Methadone and buprenorphine are first-line treatments for OUD and are the best choices for most patients; however, injectable naltrexone may be an effective alternative for select patients, such as those who are highly motivated and are experiencing homelessness.

FDA Indications:

Alcohol use disorder; OUD (relapse prevention after medically managed withdrawal).

Off-Label Uses:

Self-injurious behavior.

Dosage Forms:

- **Tablets (ReVia, [G]):** 50 mg (scored).
- **Extended-release injection (Vivitrol):** 380 mg.

Dosage Guidance:

- OUD: Start 25 mg for one day; if no withdrawal signs, increase to and maintain 50 mg/day (with food); doses >50 mg may increase risk of hepatotoxicity.
- Alcohol use disorder: Start at 50 mg QD; can increase to 100 mg QD after 12 weeks if no response.
- Injection (for opioid or alcohol use disorder): 380 mg IM (gluteal) Q4 weeks. Do not initiate therapy until patient is opioid-free for at least seven to 10 days (by urinalysis).

Monitoring: LFTs if liver disease is suspected.

Cost: Tablet: $; injection: $$$$$

Side Effects:

- Most common: Headache, nausea, somnolence, vomiting.
- Serious but rare: Black box warning regarding dose-related hepatocellular injury; the difference between apparent safe and hepatotoxic doses appears to be five-fold or less (narrow therapeutic window). Discontinue if signs/symptoms of acute hepatitis develop.

Mechanism, Pharmacokinetics, and Drug Interactions:

- Opioid antagonist.
- Metabolized primarily through non-CYP450 pathway; t ½: 4 hours (5–10 days for IM).
- No significant interactions other than avoiding use with opioids (see below).

Clinical Pearls:

- May precipitate acute withdrawal (pain, hypertension, sweating, agitation, and irritability) in opioid-using patients; ensure patient is opioid-free for at least seven to 10 days prior to initiating.
- In naltrexone-treated patients requiring emergency pain management, consider alternatives to opioids (eg, regional analgesia, non-opioid analgesics, general anesthesia). If opioid therapy is required, patients should be under the direct care of a trained anesthesia provider.
- Efficacy of oral naltrexone in alcohol use disorder (craving and relapse) is more convincing than in OUD. In OUD, craving is not decreased but euphoric effects are blocked. Monthly IM naltrexone may be more effective than oral at maintaining abstinence in OUD, without concern for daily medication adherence.
- It is recommended that patients taking naltrexone wear a medical bracelet or carry a wallet card indicating to emergency providers that they are taking naltrexone and will likely be less responsive to opioid agonist medication.

Fun Fact:

Methylnaltrexone, a closely related drug, is marketed as Relistor for the treatment of opioid-induced constipation.

Opioid Use Disorder Treatment: Psychosocial

Opioid Use Disorder: Psychosocial Approaches

Introduction

Research shows that effective opioid use disorder (OUD) treatment must include a medication such as buprenorphine, methadone, or injectable naltrexone as its main component (Amato L et al, *Cochrane Database Syst Rev* 2011;(10):CD004147). Nonetheless, psychosocial approaches can be valuable adjuncts to medications for many patients. In this fact sheet, we provide an overview of psychosocial options to consider when working with patients with OUD. Some of these treatments can be delivered by psychiatrists, while others may require referral to specialized providers. Having this information on hand is especially useful when a patient is not responding to standard treatments alone.

Psychotherapeutic Approaches

- *Motivational interviewing (MI):* MI is a patient-centered approach in which the therapist helps the patient resolve ambivalence by identifying and enhancing their intrinsic motivation to change harmful behaviors—in this case, opioid use. It can be an especially helpful approach early in treatment or with patients who are reluctant to take a medication for OUD (MOUD).

- *Cognitive behavioral therapy (CBT):* CBT focuses on helping patients identify situations that are high risk for drug use and teaches techniques for avoiding them. It teaches coping strategies for managing cravings, such as relaxation techniques, mindfulness, and distraction, as well as helping patients identify and restructure negative thought patterns. CBT works best for motivated patients who adhere to treatment, consistently practice coping skills, and will complete homework assignments.

- *12-step facilitation (TSF):* The TSF model is a semi-structured approach that connects patients to 12-step mutual-help groups, typically in the community, and encourages ongoing attendance and engagement. The group treatment approach emphasizes accountability, mutual support, and spirituality. Groups are typically peer-led and focus on building a supportive and accepting recovery community.

- *Behavioral couples therapy (BCT):* BCT includes a patient's partner in weekly sessions typically spanning three to six months. It utilizes a CBT framework in identifying risky situations, uncovering negative thought patterns, and supporting change, but does so by emphasizing communication within the couple. BCT is usually done with providers who have completed specialty training.

Behavioral Models

Contingency management (CM): CM is an approach that provides a tangible reward for abstinence. A typical model is to give patients chances to earn vouchers with monetary value or cash for not using drugs, which is verified by rapid urine drug screens. Increasing the value of the reward for consecutive negative drug screens can improve efficacy. Most evidence for CM is for stimulant use disorder, though it is being investigated for OUD as well.

Mutual-Help Groups

Various community-based organizations: Groups such as Alcoholics Anonymous and Narcotics Anonymous, best known by their acronyms AA and NA, offer free volunteer-run meetings based on the 12-step approach. Meetings are meant to foster a supportive community where participants can learn and support one another. Individual sponsorship is also usually encouraged. Attitudes and acceptance of MOUD can vary between mutual-help groups.

Harm Reduction and Opioid Use Disorder

Introduction

Harm reduction refers to a set of strategies aimed at decreasing the negative effects of drug use and other potentially harmful behaviors. As a treatment approach, harm reduction accepts that substance use is an inevitable aspect of our society. Therefore, the goal of harm reduction is to improve patient health rather than focus on full abstinence.

Examples of Harm Reduction

- *Syringe service programs (SSPs):* Formerly known as needle exchange programs, these harm reduction services provide sterile equipment for injection drug use. Early programs typically exchanged used needles and syringes for new ones, though most programs nowadays just provide sterile needles without collecting ones that have been used. They often offer additional services, including safe disposal options, wound care, overdose education, naloxone distribution, fentanyl and xylazine test strips, and referrals to substance use treatment. SSPs have been shown to decrease transmission of HIV and viral hepatitis, and they are present in at least 39 states. Your patients can locate the nearest one on the website www.harmreduction.org.

- *Fentanyl and xylazine test strips:* Originally developed for urine samples, test strips can detect fentanyl or xylazine now frequently found in street drugs. A small sample of drug is dissolved into a few milliliters of water and the strip is dipped into it. These days, almost all illicit opioids contain fentanyl, and many may contain xylazine, depending on your geographic location. Fentanyl is finding its way into other drugs such as cocaine, amphetamines, and pressed pills, so patients should be encouraged to test non-opioid drugs for the presence of fentanyl as well. Test strips are distributed by many harm reduction organizations and can be easily purchased online.

- *Supervised consumption sites:* These are clinical settings with trained medical staff where clients come to use drugs, most commonly intravenous opioids. Clients are given sterile injection equipment and staff can respond to an overdose if one were to occur. Addiction treatment, basic medical care, housing, and employment services may be offered as well. Because of legal hurdles and community opposition to such sites, there are only a few of them functioning in the US, primarily in New York City—though other large cities are planning to open new ones soon.

- *Naloxone distribution:* Great efforts have been made to increase access to naloxone, which can be used to reverse opioid overdoses. In addition to people who use opioids, naloxone is being regularly given to law enforcement, EMS workers, and friends and family of those who use drugs. Many states allow naloxone to be given without a direct prescription under legislation called a "standing order," and new over-the-counter formulations of naloxone nasal spray have recently become available.

- *Pre-exposure prophylaxis (PrEP):* Patients at high risk of contracting HIV can decrease their chance of infection by >90% if they take daily antiretroviral medication. People who engage in high-risk sexual practices or use drugs intravenously are good candidates for PrEP. The most common regimen is tenofovir disoproxil fumarate 300 mg–emtricitabine 200 mg (also known as TDF-FT), one tablet daily, to be taken as long as the patient is at high risk of infection.

How to Frame Harm Reduction Strategies With Your Patients

To keep things simple, the National Institute on Drug Abuse suggests that you give the following basic tips to all your drug-using patients:

- *Carry naloxone:* Help your patients figure out how to obtain naloxone, which is often free at pharmacies or SSPs.

- *Never use alone:* Using drugs alone increases the risk of a fatal overdose, as there may be no one present to help or administer naloxone in case of an emergency. If patients are using alone, they should connect with the National Overdose Prevention Lifeline, which is staffed with trained peers who can monitor them during use. Have patients visit www.neverusealone.com or call (877) 696-1996.

- *Go slow:* Starting with a small dose and consuming it slowly is especially important if a person has been abstinent for some time, as their tolerance may have decreased, increasing the risk of overdose. Going slow allows your patient to gauge their body's reaction to the drug and determine the "right" amount needed to achieve the desired effect.

The National Harm Reduction Coalition is an excellent resource for both general information and for information about services that are available in your area: www.harmreduction.org

How to Use Motivational Interviewing in Opioid Use Disorder

Introduction

Motivational interviewing (MI) is a therapeutic approach that focuses on a patient's own motivation and commitment to change. This method is especially useful for patients who are ambivalent about quitting. With MI, therapists aim to explore these mixed feelings and highlight the patient's reasons for wanting to get better, known as "change talk." Helping patients resolve these mixed feelings can build a strong partnership and make it easier to create a recovery plan.

MI is carried out in four steps, called Processes, each one building on the last. Here, we explain each process and offer some helpful strategies to use.

Engaging

In this first process, the goal is to establish a solid therapeutic rapport. Use nonjudgmental language and express open curiosity.

- *Active listening:* Show that you understand by using nonverbal cues (like nodding your head) and reflecting back what the patient says.
  - Patient: *"It feels impossible to get sober because every time I try to quit, I just feel so sick and start using again."*
  - Provider: *"It sounds like you want to stop using, but the withdrawals you experience are a big barrier to getting there."*
- *Open-ended questions:* Ask the patient questions like: *"How has drug use affected your life?" "What do you think about medicine to treat drug use?"*
- *Empathy and affirmation:* Offer positive reinforcement. For example: *"You've been through a lot, and I can understand why it's difficult for you to seek treatment. It's very brave of you to be here today, and I really appreciate that you made the effort."*

Focusing

The goal here is to figure out what the patient wants to achieve with treatment. Agreeing on a goal for change early on can help with planning later.

- *Agenda mapping:* Identify various possible goals and help the patient decide which is the most important for them. For example, one goal might be to start and stay on medication for opioid use disorder. A different type of goal might be one consistent with harm reduction, such as always using sterile syringes, not using alone, or not mixing opioids and stimulants.

Evoking

During this process, the provider elicits change talk, or the reasons the patient has for wanting to change their life. The goal here is to enhance change talk as much as possible and shift the conversation away from sustain talk, which are all the reasons to not make a change and instead maintain the status quo.

- *Targeted reflections:* Reflections are statements that echo back or build upon material introduced by the patient. Target your reflections so that they elicit change talk:
  - Patient: *"I know using opioids is dangerous, but stopping is so hard. It all feels so daunting."*
  - Provider: *"You mentioned that opioid use is dangerous. What are some of the dangers that you are worried about?"*

  In this case, reflecting on the dangers of opioids can provoke change talk, nudging the patient to describe why recovery is important. Avoid reflecting on how stopping is hard, because this will only cause the patient to offer more sustain talk, which is the opposite of what you want.
- *Summary statements:* Sessions are typically a mix of change talk and sustain talk. Make note of change talk statements and offer them up to the patient to remind them of all the reasons they've given to make a change:
  - *"We've touched on a lot of topics today, but what stands out to me is that you provided a lot of reasons for stopping opioids. Your friend recently passed away from an overdose, and ongoing drug use has nearly cost you your job twice. Moreover, your family is very worried about you. Does that sound right?"*

Planning

Work together with your patient to create a step-by-step action plan based on what you've talked about so far. It is important that the plan is concrete and realistic, so that the patient will be consistently moving toward their goal. Multiple small steps that are achievable will always be preferrable to big insurmountable changes.

- *SMART goals:* Patients tend to be either vague (*"I'll just use less"*) or overly ambitious (*"I'll stop cold turkey and never use again"*) when making plans for change. Instead, guide them to goals that are **S**pecific, **M**easurable, **A**ction-oriented, **R**ealistic, and **T**imely.
- *Problem solving:* Work through practical barriers that might arise while instituting a change plan: *"I'm glad you are interested in starting methadone. Do you have daily transportation to and from the clinic?" "Injectable naltrexone can be a good treatment for opioid use disorder, but it can be expensive. Have you made sure that your insurance will cover the cost?"*

How to Use Cognitive Behavioral Therapy in Opioid Use Disorder

Introduction

While psychosocial interventions are not an effective treatment for opioid use disorder (OUD) alone, smaller studies have found cognitive behavioral therapy (CBT) to be a useful adjunct for patients already on medications for OUD (Barry DT et al, *Drug Alcohol Depend* 2019;194:460–467). Here are some strategies to integrate a CBT framework into your work with patients with OUD.

1. Identify Triggers and High-Risk Situations

Help patients recognize internal and external cues that lead to opioid use. *Internal cues* are feeling states (eg, anxiety, depression). *External cues* are environmental factors (eg, financial difficulties, housing issues, family conflict).

Therapist: "Can you give me some examples of situations or feelings that might trigger your opioid use?"

Patient: "I use more when I'm stressed or when I'm around friends who also use."

Therapist: "It sounds like stress and social situations can be challenging for you. How can we develop strategies to cope with these triggers?"

If the patient is unable to identify internal or external cues, provide some examples.

Therapist: "Sometimes uncomfortable feelings, such as anxiety, depression, or anger, can lead to opioid use. Events can lead some people to use opioids as well, such as difficulty with money or being around those who use drugs. Can you identify with any of those situations?"

Identifying cues is easier for some patients than others. If they struggle coming up with cues, assure them it takes practice. The more specific the cue, the easier it will be to address.

2. Develop Coping Strategies

Use patient-generated cues to develop specific coping strategies. Tailor them closely to the patient's situation. If the patient identifies getting a call from their drug dealer as a cue, suggest blocking the dealer's number. If anxiety is an internal cue, mindfulness exercises might help. The most effective coping strategies teach patients ways to manage cravings, negative thoughts, and emotions.

Therapist: "When you experience cravings or face high-risk situations, what strategies could you use to manage those feelings? Let's brainstorm some ideas together."

Try the SMART goals framework for crafting coping strategies: **S**pecific, **M**easurable, **A**ction-oriented, **R**ealistic, **T**imely.

3. Identify Negative Thoughts

According to CBT, one's feelings are a direct result of how one interprets external events. These "automatic thoughts" form quickly and without rational input. A patient might have one occasion of opioid use and think, "I'm a total failure. I'll never get sober." This sort of negative automatic thought might make the patient feel badly and lead to further opioid use.

Learning to identify automatic thoughts, and to differentiate them from feeling states, is a central tenet of CBT. A tool that many patients and providers find useful is an **A**ctivating event, **B**elief/thought, **C**onsequence (ABC) worksheet.

Therapist: "What negative thoughts might lead you to use opioids?"

4. Challenge and Restructure Negative Thoughts

Once your patient is adept at identifying automatic thoughts, work together to challenge and restructure them. Consider adding a D column to the ABC worksheet: "**D**ispute the evidence." (See the sample ABCD worksheet in this book.)

Therapist: "Let's examine the automatic thoughts you identified and look at them rationally. Is there any actual evidence they are true? What are some other ways of seeing the situation?"

5. Relapse Prevention Planning

Develop a prevention plan. Be as collaborative as possible and refine the plan over multiple sessions (the more explicit the better):

- Write out automatic thoughts and ways the patient might restructure the thoughts when they come up
- Write out external cues and coping strategies for dealing with them

Therapist: "Let's take what we've learned so far to construct a plan minimizing the chances of going back to drug use. We should make a list of all the cues you've identified so far and write out how to cope with each so you can refer to it in the future."

Sample ABCD Worksheet for Cognitive Behavioral Therapy

Activating Event	**B**elief/Thought	**C**onsequence: Feelings & Behavior	**D**ispute the Evidence
Used once after period of abstinence	• I'm a failure • I'll never be able to stay sober • I can't do anything right, no matter how hard I try	• Embarrassment • Afraid • Wanting to avoid and isolate • Can lead to more opioid use	• Yes, I did use once, but I also was able to stay sober for 3 months. • I've had periods of sobriety before where I felt well and proud of my accomplishments. • Occasional use is a common part of recovery for many people. It doesn't mean that I'm a total failure.

Contingency Management for Opioid Use Disorder

Introduction

Contingency management (CM) is a strategy based on rewarding positive behaviors to encourage change. In the case of substance use disorders, CM often involves offering patients vouchers or cash rewards for negative urine drug screens. Rewards can also be given for attending appointments, group therapy, or counseling sessions. Securing funding for CM programs can be challenging outside of research settings, and many people still have a knee-jerk reaction against paying patients not to use drugs. Nevertheless, adding CM to medication for opioid use disorder ends up saving money as well as improving outcomes (Fairley M et al, *JAMA Psychiatry* 2021;78(7):767–777). Here are some tips for running a successful CM program.

Be Clear With Your Patients About How They Can Gain Rewards

Make sure you have objective and easy-to-measure criteria for giving rewards—such as attendance at the first intake appointment, negative urine screens, or medication adherence documented by blood levels.

Give Rewards Right Away

CM works best when rewards are given as soon as the desired behavior is shown. This means giving patients their voucher, gift card, or cash reward on the same day they provide a negative drug test.

Decide on a Voucher or an Intermittent Reward System

In a *voucher* system, patients earn a prize each time they demonstrate a desired behavior. In an *intermittent* system, patients are not necessarily rewarded each time. Instead, the desired behavior allows them to draw a ticket from a fishbowl; some tickets give prizes while others don't. Research has shown that each approach results in similar levels of abstinence (Petry NM et al, *J Consult Clin Psychol* 2005;73(6):1005). Vouchers are easier for staff to monitor but can be more costly. Intermittent systems are more cost-effective, but can be more time-consuming for staff.

Decide on a Fixed or an Escalating Reward System

In a *fixed* system, prizes remain the same over time. In an *escalating* system, prizes increase with each subsequent positive behavior. Usually, the escalating system will reset back to the beginning if the behavior is not observed (eg, if the patient has a positive urine drug screen). When paired with an intermittent CM system, this usually means that the patient is allowed to draw more tickets. Fixed systems are easier for staff to manage and for patients to understand, plus they can be more cost-efficient, but they're not as effective in promoting abstinence. Escalating systems have shown to lead to longer abstinence periods compared to fixed systems (Roll JM and Higgins ST, *Drug Alcohol Depend* 2000;59(1–2):103–109), but they can be more complicated for patients and staff.

Address Concerns

Despite the large body of evidence showing the efficacy of CM, some people object to giving cash rewards for abstinence, judging the approach to be coercive or exploitative. Make sure patients understand the rationale behind the CM approach, the details of how your program will work, and the potential benefits and risks. Emphasize that their participation is voluntary.

Think About Costs and Resources

While CM can be cost-effective in the long run, providing rewards can be expensive up front. If you're working with a limited budget, consider using lower-cost incentives like tokens that patients can trade for goods or services. Soliciting gift cards for your clinic or hospital's cafeteria or store may be a low-cost, or even free, source for prizes.

Track Progress and Adjust as Needed

Regularly review your patients' progress and adjust your CM approach as needed. This might involve changing the type or value of rewards or modifying the criteria for earning rewards. Just be sure that the conditions for doing so are laid out from the beginning.

Be Prepared for Setbacks

Just like any treatment, not all patients will be able to achieve full abstinence through a CM approach. Return to use is a common part of the recovery process. Have a plan in place to support patients who experience setbacks and consider adjusting the CM program to help them get back on track. Never treat these setbacks punitively.

Relapse Prevention Strategies

Introduction

Most patients are not able to achieve sobriety from opioids in their first attempt. In fact, many need multiple attempts before reaching a lasting recovery. Therefore, it is important to troubleshoot with your patient and develop strategies to avoid returning to use, which is often called relapse prevention. This fact sheet is designed to be used along with the "Personal Recovery Plan Template" and "Tips for Recovery" patient handouts on pages 84 and 87; we suggest reviewing the information contained here as your patient fills out the handouts in real time.

1. Recognizing Triggers

Help patients recognize feelings or situations that trigger cravings or put them at high risk of using drugs. Common triggers include HALT situations (Hungry, Angry, Lonely, Tired) and people, places, and things.

"What are some feelings that might cause you to crave opioids?"

"Who are some individuals that, when you are around them, might lead you to use opioids?"

2. Responding to Triggers, aka Coping Strategies

Work with your patient to identify coping strategies to deal with the triggers they've just identified. List strategies that the patient can utilize on their own, as well as people they can reach out to. Be as specific as possible.

"You said that feeling sad can be a trigger. How might you minimize the risk of using if you notice you feel sad?"

"Having money easily accessible is a big trigger for you. How will you keep yourself safe on payday?"

3. Dose Reduction

Medication for opioid use disorder (MOUD) is the best treatment option, but if your patient is not ready for that, a dose reduction plan can be useful. Concrete, realistic reductions can help the patient stay on track.

"Exactly which opioids are you using and how much are you taking per day? What's a realistic amount to cut back for you?"

4. Harm Reduction

After identifying a risky behavior, see if you can find a way to mitigate that risk. If the patient uses intravenously, see if they have access to sterile injection equipment. If they use alone, try to find someone to check on them.

"Some ways of using are riskier than others. Let's work together to find some ways to make your use safer."

5. Getting Help

It is important to generate a list of contacts should the patient be in a risky situation or have cravings that are difficult to manage. List individuals and organizations that the patient can reach out to, and be as specific as possible.

"It's important to have a list handy of contacts who you can call if you find yourself in a risky situation. Let's write a list together and make sure that you have up-to-date contact information for each person."

6. Medication Plan

The best strategy to prevent opioid use is to be on MOUD. If your patient is on a medication, be sure they have a thorough understanding of the dosage, how to take it, how often to take it, and how to contact the prescriber.

"I want to ensure that there aren't any questions about how to take your medication. Tell me what your understanding is."

Here are a couple strategies to keep in mind when helping your patient complete the "Tips for Recovery" handout:

Role-Play High-Risk Situations

Role-playing helps patients practice being in high-risk situations without incurring real risk. Patients can use this technique to come up with specific phrases or language that they can have at the ready.

"You mentioned that your drug dealer stopping by is a trigger for you. Let's role-play the situation and pretend that I'm your dealer coming by to make a sale. What might you say to let me know that you're not interested?"

Create a Balanced Lifestyle

Guide your patients toward using their coping strategies to build a healthy balanced lifestyle that supports long-term recovery. "White-knuckling" abstinence may work for a short time, but a sustainable sober lifestyle requires balance and self-care.

"A great way of preventing return to use is having a balanced lifestyle that promotes well-being and is sustainable over the long term. Let's discuss activities you enjoy and how to incorporate them into your daily routine."

Recovery Programs and Settings

12-Step Programs and Opioid Use Disorder

Introduction

12-step peer support groups such as Alcoholics Anonymous (AA) or Narcotics Anonymous (NA) are associated with better outcomes for those already taking medication for opioid use disorder (MOUD) (Monico LB et al, *J Subst Abuse Treat* 2015;57:89–95). Interested patients should be encouraged to attend groups, though it should not be a requirement for MOUD treatment.

In this fact sheet, we'll cover how to discuss these groups with your patients, clear up some common misconceptions, and discuss areas where traditional group approaches might diverge from the latest evidence.

Introduce the 12-Step Concept

Start by gauging interest and determining how familiar your patient is with peer support groups. If they are unfamiliar with the specifics, make sure you explain that each group has its own rules and culture. Even if your patient doesn't like the group they try first, that doesn't mean they won't like a different group. Sometimes it takes a little shopping around to find a good fit.

"Have you heard about 12-step programs like Alcoholics Anonymous or Narcotics Anonymous? They're support groups where people with substance use issues get together, share experiences, and help each other in their recovery journey. The program follows a series of steps that focus on personal growth, mutual support, and sometimes spiritual development. Many people find these groups really helpful for staying sober and preventing relapse."

Address Misconceptions

The spirituality piece can be a hang-up for some, so it's important to explain that 12-step groups do not require members to hold any specific religious belief or spiritual practice to participate. Others might think that 12-step programs are too time-intensive, lack proper confidentiality, or are even a cult.

"Sometimes people have misconceptions about 12-step programs. Just so you know, the spiritual aspect is open to interpretation; you don't have to follow any specific religious beliefs to join. Meetings are usually once a week, but you can go to as many or as few as you like. Confidentiality is really important, so everyone respects each other's privacy. And it's important for you to know that participation is always fully voluntary; you are welcome to come and go as you please."

Discuss Benefits

Talk about the potential benefits of attending 12-step meetings, such as social support, accountability, and maintaining sobriety.

"You'll get social support from peers who have gone through similar experiences and feel accountable to the group. You'll have the opportunity to learn from those who have had their own successes with sobriety, and you can teach others what you've learned. Many find that meetings help them stay focused on their recovery goals and give them a sense of community."

Encourage Attendance

Encourage your patients to check out a few meetings to see if a 12-step program is right for them. Some meetings are limited to certain groups of people: only men, only women, or meetings for those who identify as LGBTQ+.

"I recommend trying out a meeting that seems appealing, but if it doesn't work for you, just try another one. Each group is different, so you might want to try a few before deciding. Just try to be open-minded and give yourself a chance to experience what each group can offer."

Discuss Sponsorship

One major benefit of 12-step groups is the opportunity for sponsorship. Sponsors are individuals who have had a good amount of sober time under their belt, and they can serve as mentors for newer members.

"In 12-step programs, a sponsor is someone who's been in recovery longer and can help guide and support you as you work through the steps. Many people find that having a sponsor can be incredibly helpful, so I encourage you to find one."

Address Relapse Concerns

Patients may feel reluctant to keep attending group meetings if they have returned to use. Stress the importance of staying engaged with a 12-step program, especially after a return to use. It is at times like these that the program can be most helpful.

"If you do end up using again, don't hesitate to reach out to your group or sponsor. They can help you navigate the situation, learn from it, and get back on track with your recovery."

Offer Resources

Provide your patients with resources to locate 12-step meetings available in their area, such as:

- AA in-person meeting locator: https://www.aa.org/find-aa
- AA online meeting directory: https://aa-intergroup.org/meetings/
- NA in-person meeting locator: https://www.na.org/meetingsearch/
- NA virtual meetings: https://virtual-na.org

Levels of Care for Opioid Use Disorder Services

Introduction

This fact sheet offers insights into various services for opioid use disorder (OUD), highlighting their definitions, typical durations, and referral considerations to optimize patient care. They are listed in order from most to least intensive.

Withdrawal Management ("Detox")

Definition: Medically supervised programs designed to manage withdrawal symptoms; can be inpatient or outpatient.

Duration: Three to seven days.

Referral considerations:

- For patients experiencing acute withdrawal symptoms.
- Patients presenting in withdrawal should start on either buprenorphine or methadone and should generally continue these for long-term OUD treatment.
- Inpatient programs are appropriate for individuals with medical complications or those unable to abstain from opioid use for more than a few days.
- Outpatient programs are appropriate for motivated patients who are cognitively intact and have reliable transportation.

Residential Rehabilitation ("Rehab")

Definition: Nonhospital settings providing 24/7 care.

Duration: Usually 30–90 days, but can last six to 12 months.

Referral considerations:

- Well suited for patients with severe OUD who would benefit from continuous support and a stable, drug-free environment.
- Time is highly structured; patients spend most of their time on facility grounds.
- Structured schedules typically include classes, group and individual therapy, 12-step meetings, and case management.
- Rehab programs can be a great option, though they can be expensive. Some insurance plans offer limited or no coverage.
- Can be time-consuming; patients will not be able to work or spend much time with family while enrolled.
- Keep in mind that residential rehabilitation programs are not well regulated and range widely in quality. Some will not provide medication for OUD. Do research beforehand about any programs that you may be referring patients to.

Partial Hospitalization Programs (PHP)

Definition: Intensive, hospital-level care without the need for an overnight stay.

Duration: Generally two to six weeks, five to six days a week.

Referral considerations:

- Combines the intensive treatment benefits of rehab with the convenience of living at home.
- Less expensive than rehabs.
- A good option for patients with severe OUD who are otherwise highly motivated. A useful way to explain the time commitment is to compare a PHP with a full-time job.
- A potential drawback is that patients will not be in a controlled environment in the evenings.
- For patients enrolled in PHPs who are struggling with sobriety at home, consider increasing the level of care to a rehab program or arranging residence in a sober house.

Intensive Outpatient Programs (IOP)

Definition: Comprehensive therapeutic services without a requirement for an overnight stay.

Duration: Typically lasts eight to 12 weeks, with several sessions per week.

Referral considerations:

- Commonly used as a "step down" immediately following hospitalization or rehab.
- Since patients live at home and attend a few sessions weekly, this is an ideal level for patients able to maintain sobriety for several days at a time between appointments.
- Some programs have a set meeting schedule while others are flexible. Generally, IOPs have fewer sessions and are less structured, less supervised, and lower cost than PHPs.

Sober Houses

Definition: Residences providing a substance-free living environment.

Duration: Variable, ranging from several months to over a year.

Referral considerations:

- A safe and substance-free living environment.
- Ideal for patients with unstable housing or who live in an environment where drugs are easily available.
- Can serve as transitional housing while patients find more permanent living arrangements.
- Can also serve as housing while a patient attends a PHP or IOP during the day.
- Some may require 12-step program attendance or engagement with an addiction treatment provider.
- Sober houses generally do not provide formal treatment; thus, patients should also be enrolled in another form of treatment at the same time.
- Like residential rehabilitation programs, sober houses can range in quality and in how "sober" they are. Again, a bit of research before making a referral can be invaluable.

Outpatient Treatment (Ambulatory Treatment)

Definition: Clinic visits ranging from once a week to once a month.

Duration: Indefinite.

Referral considerations:

- This is the most common and least intensive treatment setting.
- Suited for patients who are stable and able to maintain sobriety.
- Patients live at home, go to work, spend time with friends and family, and regularly see their addiction providers.
- Visit schedules are agreed upon beforehand, and are usually weekly, every two weeks, or monthly.

Special Populations and Opioid Use Disorder

Managing Opioid Use Disorder in Pregnant People

Rates of opioid use disorder (OUD) and overdose deaths during pregnancy have skyrocketed in recent years. Untreated OUD is associated with many adverse outcomes, including overdose death, that can be mitigated by proper medication for opioid use disorder (MOUD) treatment. Methadone and buprenorphine have a robust evidence base, while injectable naltrexone lacks enough data to recommend during pregnancy and is not recommended.

Key Outcomes Improved by MOUD Treatment

- Mitigation of preterm birth
- Reduction of intrauterine growth restriction
- Prevention of maternal cardiac arrest
- Lowering of placental abruption
- Reduction of comorbid substance use
- Prevention of fatal and non-fatal overdose

Treatment Recommendations

- Avoid withdrawal: Opioid withdrawal can lead to catecholamine surges, inducing uterine contractions, reducing placental blood flow, and potentially causing fetal hypoxia, preterm birth, and fetal demise.
- Both methadone and buprenorphine have been proven safe and effective in pregnancy, with differing pros and cons; neither is universally superior.
- Methadone is associated with a lower dropout rate over the course of pregnancy when compared to buprenorphine.
- Buprenorphine results in less severe neonatal opioid withdrawal syndrome and shorter post-delivery hospital stays compared to methadone.

Prescribing Methadone in Pregnancy

- Initiate treatment in the hospital setting.
- Begin with a small first dose (5–10 mg) unless the patient is in withdrawal. Give another 5–10 mg if withdrawal symptoms develop.
- In cases of opioid withdrawal, start with a higher dose (20–30 mg) and add 5–10 mg every three to six hours until withdrawal is relieved, up to a maximum of 50 mg in 24 hours. Treat residual withdrawal using typical symptomatic treatment (see "Managing Opioid Withdrawal in the Inpatient Setting" fact sheet).
- While in the hospital, daily methadone dose can be increased by 5–10 mg until withdrawal and cravings are adequately treated.
- Once stable, arrange follow-up at a federally recognized opioid treatment program.
- Adjust dosage more slowly in outpatient settings; weekly increase should not exceed 10 mg per day.
- Doses may need to be higher during pregnancy (>120 mg/day), particularly in the last trimester due to increased metabolism. Potentially split into twice-daily dosing for a steadier plasma concentration.

Prescribing Buprenorphine in Pregnancy

- Buprenorphine induction after 24 weeks gestation should be done in the hospital. This is the gestational age after which routine fetal monitoring is feasible.
- Outpatient induction can be considered before 24 weeks of gestation with immediate ER evaluation if precipitated withdrawal develops.
- Utilize typical induction procedure (see "How to Discuss and Initiate Buprenorphine" fact sheet for further details):
  - Give an initial dose of 2–4 mg once Clinical Opiate Withdrawal Scale score >8. Give additional doses of 2–4 mg every two to four hours for a total dose of 8–12 mg in the first 24 hours.
  - Give the total amount received on day 1 as a single dose on the morning of day 2. Continue to give additional doses for residual symptoms up to a total daily dose of 16 mg.
  - Repeat on day 3 up to 24 mg, which is the usual maximum daily dose.
- Dose adjustments of buprenorphine during pregnancy are typically less frequent than with methadone.
- Either buprenorphine monoproduct or buprenorphine/naloxone combination can be used in pregnancy. The monoproduct has historically been favored due to potential risks of fetal naloxone exposure, but data support the safe use of the combination product during pregnancy (Link HM et al, *Am J Obstet Gynecol* 2020;2(3):100179).

Postpartum

- Some patients on methadone may need their dose lowered after delivery, though others will do better by remaining on the high dose reached during pregnancy (Link et al, 2020). Monitor your patient carefully for signs of oversedation and gradually lower the dose if necessary.
- Encourage continuation of treatment after delivery; MOUD decreases overdose mortality tenfold six months postpartum compared to those not on treatment (Schiff DM et al, *Obstet Gynecol* 2018;132(2):466–474).
- Promote breastfeeding in patients who are not using illicit substances other than opioids, as it lowers the incidence and severity of neonatal opioid withdrawal syndrome.

Other Considerations

- Pregnancy can be a touchpoint for additional supportive services like prenatal care, nutrition counseling, housing assistance, and case management.
- Patient concerns about infant foster care placement due to MOUD should be addressed. In reality, MOUD treatment increases the likelihood of the infant being discharged home with their biological parent (Singelton R et al, *J Addict Med* 2022;16(6):e366–e373).

Neonatal Opioid Withdrawal Syndrome: Recognition and Management

Clinical Presentation and Diagnosis

Neonatal opioid withdrawal syndrome (NOWS), sometimes used interchangeably with the term neonatal abstinence syndrome (NAS), results from prenatal opioid exposure. Withdrawal symptoms typically surface anywhere from 72 hours to seven days post-birth, and though typically not fatal, NOWS is distressing and can lead to prolonged hospitalization of both the infant and the mother. NOWS severity is measured by the Finnegan Neonatal Abstinence Scoring System.

Symptoms include:

- Poor and fragmented sleep
- Tremors
- Sweating
- Congestion
- Fever
- Yawning
- Mottled skin
- Irritability
- High-pitched crying
- Gassiness, vomiting, diarrhea
- Poor feeding

Management and Treatment

Before delivery

- Educate your pregnant patients with substance use disorders about the risks of NOWS and the importance of prenatal care and substance use treatment.
- A risk of NOWS is not a reason to wean pregnant patients off medication for opioid use disorder (MOUD). In fact, keeping pregnant patients on MOUD reduces risks of preterm labor, illicit opioid use, and a host of infant adverse outcomes (Krans EE et al, *Addiction* 2021;116(12):3504–3514).
- Methadone and buprenorphine are both effective MOUDs during pregnancy, though methadone is associated with more severe NOWS.

Non-pharmacological interventions

- Rooming-in and parental involvement: Promotes bonding and early NOWS symptom recognition.
- Swaddling, skin-to-skin contact, and breastfeeding: Calms infant, strengthens bonding, and reduces NOWS severity.

Pharmacological interventions

The aim of pharmacological treatment is symptom reduction, enabling the infant to feed, regulate movements, and interact with caregivers. Severity is tracked every 3–4 hours using the Finnegan scoring system, and medication doses are given if a threshold is met, usually two consecutive scores ≥12 or three consecutive scores ≥8 (Kockerlakota P, *Pediatrics* 2014 Aug;134(2):e547–e561). Various modifications of the Finnegan scoring system are out there, and most institutions will have their own preferred version. See the example below (see page 74) for a typical scoring system.

First-line medications:

- *Morphine:* Typical dosing is 0.04–0.16 mg/kg PO every three to four hours. Adjust dose based on infant weight and symptom severity. Taper the dose by 10%–20% every 48–72 hours as tolerated.
- *Methadone:* Initial dosing is 0.05–0.1 mg/kg PO every six to eight hours. Taper the dose by 10% every two to three days, depending on infant response and symptom severity.
- Buprenorphine is typically not used because of challenges with sublingual administration and the possibility of precipitated withdrawal.

Second-line medications:

- *Clonidine:* Alpha-2 adrenergic agonist used alongside morphine or methadone. Initial dose is 0.5–0.75 mcg/kg every three hours and can be increased to 1 mcg/kg every three hours. Taper dose by 10% every one to two days.
- *Phenobarbital:* Barbiturates can be used in severe NOWS or benzodiazepine exposure. Loading dose is 10–20 mg/kg ×1 dose, followed by 2.5 mg/kg twice daily. Dose is tapered by 10%–15% every two to three days depending on infant response.

Example of a Modified Finnegan Neonatal Abstinence Score

Cry	Normal = 0 Excessive high pitched <5 mins = 2 Continuous high pitched >5 mins = 3	
Sleep	Normal = 1 Sleeps <3 hrs after feeding = 1 Sleeps <2 hrs after feeding = 2 Sleeps <1 hr after feeding = 3	
Moro	Normal = 0 Hyperactive = 2 Very hyperactive = 3	
Tremor	None = 0 Mild if disturbed = 1 Mod-severe if disturbed = 2 Mild undisturbed = 3 Mod-severe undisturbed = 4	
Muscle tone	Normal = 0 Increased = 1	
Myclonic jerk	None = 0 Present = 1	
Seizure	None = 0 Present = 5	
Sweating	None = 0 Present = 1	
Fever	None = 0 37.2–38.3°C (99.0–100.9°F) = 1 >38.3°C (>100.9°F) = 2	
Yawning	Normal = 0 >3–4 times over interval of scoring = 1	
Skin mottling	None = 0 Present = 1	
Congestion	None = 0 Present = 1	
Sneezing	Normal = 0 >3–4 times over interval of scoring = 1	
Nasal flaring	None = 0 Present = 2	
Respirations	Normal = 0 >60 per min w/o retractions = 1 >60 per min w retractions = 2	
Sucking	Normal = 0 Excessive = 1	
Feeding	Normal = 0 Infrequent or uncoordinated = 2	
Regurgitation	Normal = 0 Twice or more during/post feeding = 2	
Projectile vomiting	None = 0 Present = 3	
Stool	Normal = 0 Loose = 2 Watery = 3	
		TOTAL =

Perioperative Management of Patients on Medications for Opioid Use Disorder

Introduction

Medications for opioid use disorder (MOUD) can complicate pain control during and after surgery. While there are no universally adopted protocols for managing MOUD in the perioperative period, there are nonetheless helpful guidelines to consider for your patients preparing for surgery.

General Principles

- Communicate and collaborate closely with the surgical and anesthesia teams
- Always optimize non-opioid medications for pain control
- Discuss whether regional anesthesia can be used for your patient's procedure
- Whenever possible, keep your patient in a controlled environment (ie, inpatient) for any period in which they are not on full-dose MOUD
- Patients not on MOUD may be particularly susceptible to pain and are at increased risk of returning to use in the postop period

Methadone

As a full agonist, methadone will not block the effects of other concurrently administered agonists during or after surgery and therefore does not need adjustment (Harrison TK et al, *Anesthesiology Clin* 2018;36(3):345–359).

- Continue home dose throughout the perioperative period; communicate and coordinate planning with methadone clinic
- Use short-acting opioids for additional pain control for ≤7 days after surgery
- Don't increase methadone for pain control since doses can "stack" due to methadone's long half-life
- If possible, split methadone to BID or TID for the immediate postop period
- Switch to IV if the patient can't take PO; reduce dose to one-half to two-thirds

Buprenorphine

Concerns that buprenorphine complicates pain management during the perioperative period are likely exaggerated (Kornfeld H and Manfredi L, *Am J Ther* 2010;17:523–528). Nonetheless, the tight receptor affinity and partial agonism of buprenorphine does mean it could theoretically interfere with other opioids used during and after surgery. We recommend adjusting the buprenorphine dose only in cases when severe postop pain is expected; the surgical and anesthesia teams can help you determine the level of expected pain for a given procedure if you aren't sure.

- If mild or moderate postop pain is expected, continue buprenorphine unchanged
- For major surgeries when severe postop pain is expected:
  - Give full buprenorphine dose the day before surgery
  - Give a small dose (4–8 mg) preoperatively
  - Restart full dose on the day after surgery
- Use short-acting opioids for additional pain control for ≤7 days after surgery

Naltrexone

As an opioid blocker, naltrexone can interfere with the function of opioid analgesic medications. Ideally, the medication should be stopped prior to surgery.

- Oral naltrexone should be stopped for two to three days before surgery
- Extended-release injectable naltrexone should be held for 30 days before surgery
- Patients on naltrexone do not have opioid tolerance, so they may be very sensitive to opioids
- Naltrexone can be restarted once patients are off opioid analgesics for seven to 10 days

Patient Handouts

BUPRENORPHINE Fact Sheet for Patients

Generic Name: Buprenorphine (byoo-pre-NOR-feen)

Brand Names: Brixadi, Bunavail, Sublocade, Suboxone, Subutex, Zubsolv

What Does It Treat?

This medication is used to help manage moderate to severe opioid use disorder. It is also used to provide relief from moderate to severe pain.

How Does It Work?

Buprenorphine is a drug that helps lessen withdrawal symptoms and cravings for opioids. Using it is linked to reduced illicit opioid use and deaths due to overdoses, as well as lower rates of death from cancer, suicide, alcohol-related issues, and heart diseases.

How Do I Take It?

Buprenorphine can be taken as a tablet or film under the tongue, as a film placed on the inside of the cheek, or as a weekly or monthly injection under the skin. Tablets under the tongue can take up to 10 minutes to fully dissolve, while films can take up to two minutes to dissolve. Allowing the medication to fully dissolve ensures that your body fully absorbs it. After the medication is dissolved, rinse your mouth with water and avoid brushing your teeth or eating for an hour. If the taste is not to your liking, you can chew a sugar-free peppermint before and after taking the tablet. Injections are administered at a doctor's office or pharmacy, not at home.

How Long Will I Take It?

Stopping buprenorphine can lead to an increased risk of death from opioid overdose, so many people continue to take it indefinitely. The duration of treatment varies, but it's generally recommended to take it for at least 12 months, as this duration has been linked with better results. Do not stop taking it on your own; discuss with your provider if you'd like to consider stopping it.

What if I Miss a Dose?

If you forget to take a dose, take it as soon as you remember, unless it's nearly time for your next dose. In that case, skip the missed dose. Do not take a double dose to make up for the missed one.

What Are Possible Side Effects?

- Most common: Constipation, headaches, trouble sleeping, nausea, anxiety.
- Serious but rare: Liver inflammation (hepatitis), abnormal heart rhythm (QT prolongation).

What Else Should I Know?

- It's important to follow your doctor's instructions when taking buprenorphine to ensure it's used safely and to prevent misuse.
- Avoid taking other opioids or central nervous system depressants, like benzodiazepines, while you're on buprenorphine.
- Make sure to inform your healthcare providers that you're taking this medication. Consider carrying a card in your wallet or something similar to indicate you're on this medication.
- Some forms of buprenorphine include another medication called naloxone. The combination is often used because it is more widely available and may be less likely to be misused. If you're pregnant or have a negative reaction to naloxone, you might be prescribed buprenorphine alone.

METHADONE (Methadose) Fact Sheet for Patients

Generic Name: Methadone (METH-uh-doan)

Brand Name: Methadose

What Does It Treat?

This medication is used to help manage moderate to severe opioid use disorder. It is also used to provide relief from moderate to severe pain.

How Does It Work?

Methadone is a drug that helps lessen withdrawal symptoms and cravings for opioids. Using it is linked to reduced illicit opioid use and deaths due to overdoses, as well as lower rates of death from cancer, suicide, alcohol-related issues, and heart diseases.

How Do I Take It?

Methadone comes as a tablet when used for pain, and as an oral solution when used for opioid use disorder. For opioid use disorder, it is typically taken once daily. You'll start with a lower dose that will be increased depending on your symptoms.

Where Do I Get It?

Methadone for the treatment of opioid use disorder must be dispensed from a federally regulated facility called an opioid treatment program, commonly known as a "methadone clinic." Initially, you'll visit the clinic six days a week. As your treatment progresses, you may be able to take some doses home, and your visits may drop to once a week.

How Long Will I Take It?

Stopping methadone can lead to an increased risk of death from opioid overdose, so many people continue to take it indefinitely. Do not stop taking it on your own; discuss with your provider if you'd like to consider stopping it.

What if I Miss a Dose?

If you forget to take a dose, take it as soon as you remember, unless it's nearly time for your next dose. In that case, skip the missed dose. Do not take a double dose to make up for the missed one.

What Are Possible Side Effects?

- Most common: Constipation, dizziness, sleepiness, nausea, sweating.
- Serious but rare: Changes in heart rhythm (QT prolongation), severe respiratory depression.

What Else Should I Know?

- Methadone may interact with other medicines you're taking, so be sure to tell your healthcare provider about all your medications.
- Methadone is a tightly regulated substance and must be dispensed according to specific rules. For more information, check with your local methadone treatment facility.
- Since methadone builds up in your body with each dose, you might need to reduce your dose after three to five days to prevent potential side effects.

NALTREXONE (ReVia, Vivitrol) Fact Sheet for Patients

Generic Name: Naltrexone (nal-TREX-own)

Brand Names: ReVia (tablet), Vivitrol (injection)

What Does It Treat?

Naltrexone is used in the treatment of alcohol and opioid use disorder.

How Does It Work?

For treating opioid use disorder, naltrexone injection blocks opioids from getting into your brain. It also helps to curb cravings, leading to less opioid use.

How Do I Take It?

Naltrexone comes as a pill (ReVia) or an extended-release injection (Vivitrol). For opioid use disorder, only the injectable version has proven effective. To start naltrexone, you need to be opioid-free for a week to 10 days—taking naltrexone any sooner could trigger opioid withdrawal. Once you're free of opioids, naltrexone is given as an injection in the buttock every three to four weeks.

Where Do I Get It?

Your healthcare provider can prescribe naltrexone. The injection is typically given at the doctor's office, in a pharmacy, in a hospital, or at a treatment facility. Sometimes, a visiting nurse can administer it at your home.

What Are Possible Side Effects?

- Most common: Nausea, headache, dizziness, anxiety, fatigue, sleep difficulties.
- Serious but rare: Liver damage and allergic reactions (eg, rash, swelling, difficulty breathing).

What Else Should I Know?

- Naltrexone can interact with other medications, so be sure to let your healthcare provider know about all the medicines you're taking.
- Avoid using naltrexone if you're currently using opioids or if you have severe liver disease or liver failure.
- Before starting naltrexone, inform your healthcare provider if you have any history of liver issues or other medical problems.
- Consider carrying an ID card or wearing a medical alert bracelet indicating that you're taking naltrexone. This could be lifesaving information in an emergency.

NALMEFENE (Opvee) Fact Sheet for Patients

Generic Name: Nalmefene (nal-muh-FEEN)

Brand Name: Opvee

What Does It Treat?
Nalmefene is used to reverse opioid overdose in emergency situations.

How Does It Work?
Nalmefene is an opioid blocker that quickly counteracts the life-threatening effects of an opioid overdose by binding to the same receptors in the brain as opioids, temporarily reversing their effects.

How Do I Use It?
- Opvee comes in a nasal spray form. During an overdose, a person nearby can spray it into one nostril, wait two to three minutes, and, if needed, repeat the process in the other nostril. This can continue every few minutes until the person wakes up.
- Nalmefene also comes as an injection that can be administered into a vein, into a muscle, or just under the skin.
- Since some opioids may stick around in the body longer than nalmefene, it's crucial to get emergency medical help immediately to prevent another overdose episode. If the person isn't breathing, start mouth-to-mouth resuscitation until professional help arrives.

Where Do I Get It?
Opvee is available through a prescription and is dispensed at a pharmacy.

What Are Possible Side Effects?
- There are very few or no side effects if there are no opioids in your system. If you do have opioids in your system, nalmefene can cause withdrawal symptoms.
- Most common: Symptoms of opioid withdrawal, including body aches, sweating, runny nose, sneezing, goosebumps, yawning, weakness, shivering or trembling, nervousness, restlessness or irritability, diarrhea, nausea or vomiting, abdominal cramps, increased blood pressure, and rapid heartbeat.

What Else Should I Know?
- Tell those around you that you have nalmefene, and make sure they know how to recognize an overdose and how to use the medication.
- After using nalmefene, immediately call 911 and avoid using more opioids.
- Nalmefene doesn't last as long as some opioids, so overdose symptoms may return after the initial improvement. Always seek medical attention after using an emergency dose of nalmefene.

NALOXONE (Kloxxado, Narcan Nasal Spray, RiVive, Zimhi) Fact Sheet for Patients

Generic Name: Naloxone (nal-OX-one)

Brand Names: Kloxxado, Narcan Nasal Spray, RiVive, Zimhi

What Does It Treat?

Naloxone is used to reverse opioid overdose in emergency situations.

How Does It Work?

Naloxone is an opioid blocker that quickly counteracts the life-threatening effects of an opioid overdose by binding to the same receptors in the brain as opioids, temporarily reversing their effects.

How Do I Use It?

- Naloxone, Kloxxado, and RiVive come in a nasal spray form. During an overdose, a person nearby can spray it into one nostril, wait two to three minutes, and, if needed, repeat the process in the other nostril. This can continue every few minutes until the person wakes up.
- Naloxone also comes as an injection that can be administered either into a muscle or just under the skin.
- Since most opioids stick around in the body longer than naloxone, it's crucial to get emergency medical help immediately to prevent another overdose episode. If the person isn't breathing, start mouth-to-mouth resuscitation until professional help arrives.

Where Do I Get It?

Naloxone is available through a prescription, can be dispensed at a pharmacy without a prescription, or can be sold over the counter. Various organizations that aim to reduce harm from drug use also distribute naloxone, often for free. You can find such places on the National Harm Reduction Coalition's website (www.harmreduction.org).

What Are Possible Side Effects?

- There are very few or no side effects if there are no opioids in your system. If you do have opioids in your system, naloxone can cause withdrawal symptoms.
- Most common: Symptoms of opioid withdrawal, including body aches, sweating, runny nose, sneezing, goosebumps, yawning, weakness, shivering or trembling, nervousness, restlessness or irritability, diarrhea, nausea or vomiting, abdominal cramps, increased blood pressure, and rapid heartbeat.

What Else Should I Know?

- Tell those around you that you have naloxone, and make sure they know how to recognize an overdose and how to use the medication.
- After using naloxone, immediately call 911 and avoid using more opioids.
- Naloxone doesn't last as long as most opioids, so overdose symptoms may return after the initial improvement. Always seek medical attention after using an emergency dose of naloxone.

Personal Recovery Plan Template Fact Sheet for Patients

Fill out this sheet with your provider in order to put together a personal recovery plan. Working on this plan will help you come up with coping strategies, identify supports, define your triggers, and help you maintain healthy routines. It also promotes accountability, goal setting, and self-reflection. Once completed, print out a hard copy so that you can have it available whenever you might need it.

Triggers That Put Me at Risk for Using

(Example: Going home after work to have unstructured time makes me more likely to use.)

1. _____
2. _____
3. _____

How I Will Address Each Trigger

(Example: Each day after work, I will go to the gym or to a 12-step meeting.)

1. _____
2. _____
3. _____

Ways I Will Increase My Self-Care

(Example: I will be sure to take buprenorphine as directed every day and keep appointments with my therapist.)

1. _____
2. _____
3. _____

Coping Skills I Will Learn or Improve Upon and How I Will Do This

(Example: I will meet with my therapist weekly and practice relaxation techniques every day.)

1. _____
2. _____
3. _____

My Relapse Prevention Strategies

(Example: I will program my sponsor's number into my speed dial and call as soon as I feel an opioid craving.)

1. _____
2. _____
3. _____

Additional Commitments to Help Me Stick to My Plan

(Example: I will stay sober so that I can be there for my grandchildren as they grow up.)

1. _____
2. _____
3. _____

(Adapted from a template provided by American Addiction Centers: www.recovery.org/pro/articles/developing-your-personal-recovery-plan-template-included/)

Opioid Overdose Overview Fact Sheet for Patients

Introduction

Opioids can cause a bad and potentially fatal reaction (overdose) that makes your breathing slow or even stop, which can be fatal. Opioids include prescriptions such as hydrocodone, oxycodone, morphine, codeine, and hydromorphone. Other opioids are heroin and fentanyl, which can be obtained illicitly or may contaminate street drugs like cocaine, methamphetamine, or counterfeit pills.

How to Avoid an Accidental Opioid Overdose

- Only take medicine prescribed to you and don't take more than prescribed.
- Don't mix opioids with alcohol, benzodiazepines (Xanax, Ativan, Klonopin, Valium), or medicines that make you sleepy.
- Don't use opioids while alone. If you do use alone, call the Never Use Alone hotline at (877) 696-1996 prior to using.
- Don't use opioids from an unknown source.
- If you haven't taken opioids for some time, start with a very small "tester dose." It is likely that you won't need to take as much as before.
- Store your opioids in a secure place and dispose of unused medications to minimize risk of others overdosing.
- Have naloxone on hand and teach your family and friends how to respond to an overdose.

How to Respond to an Opioid Overdose

A Patient-Centered Guide to Managing an Opioid Overdose	

STEP 1
Assess
	• Try to arouse the person by loudly calling their name and giving them a firm shake. If they don't wake up, vigorously rub your knuckles into the sternum (the breastbone in the middle of the chest) or pinch the ear lobes to wake them up.
	• Look for the classic signs of an opioid overdose:
	  – Slow breathing
	  – Not awakening
	  – Very small pupils
	• If they remain unresponsive, move on to Step 2.

STEP 2 Call 911	• Opioid overdoses need immediate medical attention. • Call 911 right away (say "someone is unresponsive and not breathing"; give clear address and location).
STEP 3 Administer naloxone	• Administer a dose of naloxone as early as possible. • If the person doesn't respond within two to three minutes, give a second dose of naloxone.
STEP 4 Support breathing	• If the person doesn't have a pulse, CPR will be needed. • If the person isn't breathing but still has a pulse, perform rescue breathing by giving one breath every five seconds. • Do not leave the person alone. Wait for emergency responders to arrive; while waiting, follow their instructions, which may include placing the person into the recovery position: Hand under chin to keep mouth open Leg bent to support position Arm bent to prevent rolling over
STEP 5 Monitor response	• Because naloxone only lasts for a short time, overdose symptoms may return. • Ensure the person does not use more opioids after naloxone revival. They may be in withdrawal, but naloxone will prevent opioids from relieving symptoms and they will risk overdosing again once naloxone is eliminated from their body. • It is critical that the person be transferred to the emergency department, even if there is a full revival.

Subjective Opiate Withdrawal Scale (SOWS) Fact Sheet for Patients

Introduction

The Subjective Opiate Withdrawal Scale (SOWS) is a scale that can be used to define the severity of opioid withdrawal symptoms at home without the involvement of a health care provider. This scale can be used at home when starting buprenorphine. Once you start experiencing withdrawal, score your symptoms every few hours—you should be ready for your first buprenorphine dose once your total score adds up to 10 or higher.

Patient Instructions

At the top of the first column below, write in today's date and time, and in the rows underneath, write in a number from 0 to 4 corresponding to how you feel about each symptom *right now*.

Scale: 0 = not at all, 1 = a little, 2 = moderately, 3 = quite a bit, 4 = extremely.

Date					
Time					
Symptom	Score	Score	Score	Score	Score
I feel anxious					
I feel like yawning					
I am perspiring					
My eyes are teary					
I have goosebumps					
I am shaking					
I have hot flashes					
My bones and muscles ache					
I feel restless					
I feel nauseous					
I feel like vomiting					
My muscles twitch					
I have stomach cramps					
I feel like using now					
TOTAL					

Mild withdrawal = score of 1–10

Moderate withdrawal = score of 11–20

Severe withdrawal = score of 21–30

Source: Adapted from Handelman L et al, *Am J Drug Alcohol Abuse* 1987;13(3):293–308.

Tips for Recovery Fact Sheet for Patients

Introduction

Use this sheet to write out specific situations that might put you at risk of using opioids and what to do about each one. Filling out the sheet with your provider can be a great way of collaborating on a recovery plan. Once you finish, print out a hard copy so it is always accessible, and keep it up to date.

Recognizing and Responding to Triggers

Triggers that can lead to drug use
List feelings (eg, anger, sadness) and situations (eg, "My dealer comes by," "I visit my friends who offer me drugs")

Coping strategies	
Strategies to use on my own (eg, mindfulness exercises, going for a walk, listening to music)	Supports that I can reach out to; include contact info (eg, Jill, friend, 555-1212; Jack, sponsor, 555-8989)

Staying Safe

Dose reduction	
How much you are currently using; be specific (eg, one bundle of heroin fentanyl IV daily)	Reduction plan (eg, one less pill or one less dose each day)

Harm reduction	
Risky behaviors (eg, sharing needles)	How to be safer (eg, only using sterile needles from the syringe exchange)

Where to Get Help

Name of support	How to contact (enter contact info below)
Suicide and Crisis Lifeline	Dial 988
Alcoholics Anonymous	
Narcotics Anonymous	
Clinic name	
Therapist name	
Nearest hospital	

Medication Plan

Name of medication (eg, methadone, buprenorphine, injectable naltrexone)	Dose (number of milligrams and frequency)	Prescriber name and contact

Appendix

Opioid Use Disorder Medications

Generic Name (Brand Name) Year FDA Approved (Rx status) *[G] denotes generic availability*	Relevant FDA Indication(s)	Available Strengths (mg)	Usual Dosage Range (mg)
Buprenorphine [G] (Belbuca, Buprenex, Butrans) 2002 (Schedule III)	Opioid use	2, 8 SL 0.075, 0.15, 0.3, 0.45, 0.6, 0.75, 0.9 buccal film (Belbuca, [G]) (used for pain) 0.3 mg/mL injection (Buprenex, [G]) (used for pain) 5, 7.5, 10, 15, 20 mcg/hr patch (Butrans) (used for pain)	8–16 QD SL
Buprenorphine extended-release injection (Sublocade) 2017 (Schedule III)	Opioid use	100, 300	300 mg SC monthly ×2 doses, then 100 mg or 300 mg monthly
Buprenorphine extended-release injection (Brixadi) 2023 (Schedule III)	Opioid use	8, 16, 24, 32 (weekly) 64, 96, 128 (monthly)	8–32 SC weekly 64–128 SC monthly
Buprenorphine and naloxone [G] (Bunavail, Suboxone, Zubsolv) 2002 (Schedule III) Generic available for 2/0.5, 8/2 mg SL tablets and SL film strips only	Opioid use	2.1/0.3, 4.2/0.7, 6.3/1 buccal film (Bunavail) 2/0.5, 4/1, 8/2, 12/3 SL film strip (Suboxone, [G]) 2/0.5, 8/2 SL tablet (generic only) 0.7/0.18, 1.4/0.36, 2.9/0.71, 5.7/1.4, 8.6/2.1, 11.4/2.9 SL tablet (Zubsolv)	8–24 QD
Clonidine [G] (Catapres, Kapvay) 1974 (Rx)	Opioid use (decreases withdrawal symptoms)	0.1, 0.2, 0.3 IR tablet 0.1, 0.2 ER tablet 0.1, 0.2, 0.3 mg/day patch	0.1–0.2 Q4–Q6 hours PRN (IR tablet)
Lofexidine (Lucemyra) 2018 (Rx)	Opioid use (decreases withdrawal symptoms)	0.18	3–4 tablets QID, then taper
Methadone [G] (Dolophine, Methadose) 1947 (Schedule II)	Opioid use	5, 10, 40 10 mg/mL, 10 mg/5 mL, 5 mg/5 mL oral liquid	20–120 QD
Nalmefene [G] (Opvee) 1995 (injectable), 2023 (intranasal) (Rx)	Opioid use (emergency opioid overdose rescue)	2.7 mg/0.1 mL (intranasal) 2 mg/2 mL (injection)	×1; may repeat every 2–5 minutes (intranasal) 0.5 mg ×1; may repeat with 1 mg 2–5 minutes later (injection)
Naloxone [G] (Kloxxado, Narcan Nasal Spray, RiVive, Zimhi) 2015 (intranasal) (Rx/OTC)	Opioid use (emergency opioid overdose rescue)	3 mg/0.1 mL intranasal (RiVive) 4 mg/0.1 mL intranasal (Narcan) 8 mg/0.1 mL intranasal (Kloxxado) 5 mg/0.5 mL intramuscular or subcutaneous (Zimhi)	×1; may repeat every 2–3 minutes
Naltrexone ER (Vivitrol) 2006 (Rx)	Opioid use (blocks opioid effects)	380	380 Q4 weeks

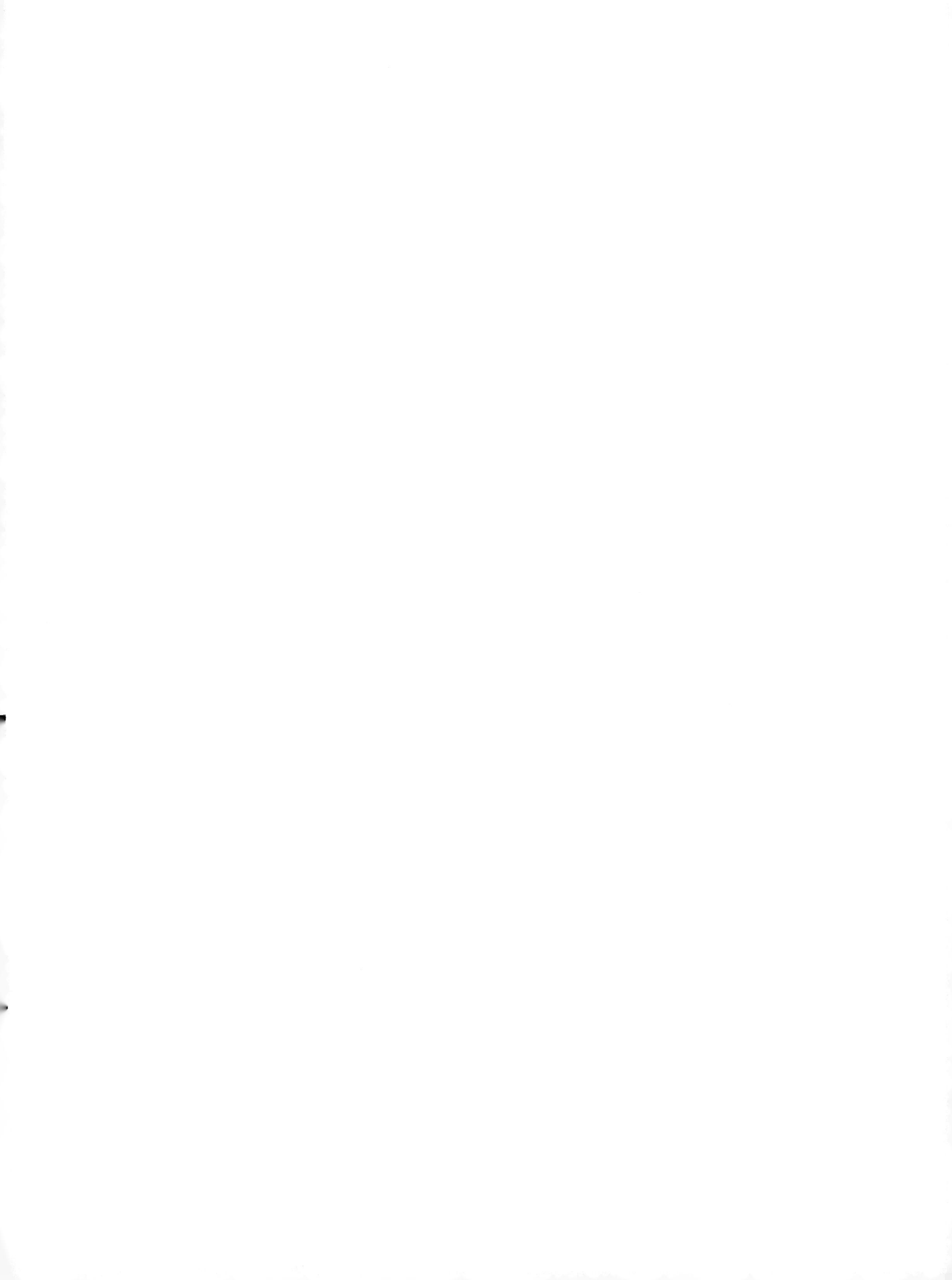